HOW THE RICH GET THIN

HOW THE RICH GET THIN

Park Avenue's Top Diet Doctor

Reveals the Secrets to

Losing Weight and Feeling Great

JANA KLAUER, M.D.

ST. MARTIN'S PRESS ⚏ NEW YORK

www.stmartins.com

Design by Patrice Sheridan

LIBRARY OF CONGRESS CATALOGING-IN-PUBLICATION DATA

Klauer, Jana.
    How the rich get thin : Park Avenue's top diet doctor reveals the secrets to losing weight and feeling great / Jana Klauer.—1st ed.
        p.   cm.
    Includes bibliographical references (p. 229) and index (p. 259).
    ISBN 0-312-34038-9
    EAN 978-0-312-34038-4
    1. High-calcium diet.   2. High-calcium diet—Recipes.   3. Reducing exercises. I. Title.

RM237.56.K53   2006
613.2'5—dc22   2005052044

First Edition: January 2006

10 9 8 7 6 5 4 3 2 1

To Erika, because you helped when I needed you most

NOTE TO THE READER

The information contained in this book should by no means be construed as a substitute for the advice of a qualified medical professional, who should always be consulted before beginning any new health, diet, or exercise program. If you are pregnant or nursing, or taking any kind of prescription medications, or are under the care of a physician, please consult with your physician before starting any health, diet, or exercise program and for optimum dosage requirements of all vitamins, nutrients, and supplements.

CONTENTS

ACKNOWLEDGMENTS

.

I would like to acknowledge the influence and thank the individuals who have shaped my clinical practice and this book.

At the Mount Sinai School of Medicine, I was particularly influenced by Dr. Edward Ronan, a gifted teacher of biochemistry and pharmacology. Michael J. Klein, M.D., and Robert Phelps, M.D., are both pathologists and enabled me to understand the working of the body on a microscopic level. John Rowe, M.D., past president of Mount Sinai, was an inspiring teacher and healer.

The faculty of the Columbia University School of Human Nutrition presented nutritional topics with thoroughness and insight. I would like to thank David Talmadge, Ph.D., Sharon Akabas, R.D., Ph.D., and Maudene Nelson, R.D., for teaching me about human nutrition.

At the New York Obesity Research Center of St. Luke's Roosevelt Hospital, the legendary F. Xavier Pi-Sunyer, M.D., generously taught me about obesity. Dr. Pi-Sunyer was one of the first individuals to recognize obesity as a disease. It was an honor to be a part of his great institution. Carol Boozer, Ph.D., was a patient mentor in the intricacies of conducting clinical trials.

Louis Aronne, M.D., allowed me to manage his clinical trial, introduced me to treatment of obesity, and encouraged me to enter the field of medical weight reduction. It was through his guidance that I had the courage to start my own practice.

Marianne J. Legato, M.D., is an inspiring physician who I have been delighted to work with for the last four years.

My agent, Richard Curtis, deserves credit for taking a new writer under his wing and introducing me to St. Martin's.

Sally Richardson, the publisher at St. Martin's, and Elizabeth Beier, my talented editor, believed in the book at the first presentation. These dynamic women have my deepest gratitude. The wonderful genius Wendy Lewis, who helped me arrive at the finished product, was invaluable. John Murphy, head of publicity, enthusiastically supported the book. Lisa Senz was a dynamo in her creative marketing ideas. The entire staff at St. Martin's marketing, design, production, and sales gets a round of applause from me.

My trainer, Joe Masiello, of Focus Fitness, kept me strong through our 6:00 A.M. "get-togethers."

I also want to thank S.P.L. (you know who you are) because you enabled me to change.

Lastly, how can I adequately thank my brilliant, handsome, and wonderful husband, Gerold Klauer, who had the chutzpah to put up with four years of medical school, four years of clerkship, two years of master's degree study, and a one-year fellowship. He is a rock and deserves a medal! Our children, Matthew and Erika, are a source of joy and pride. Their support and love mean everything to me.

INTRODUCTION

Park Avenue. These two words conjure up images of wealth, privilege, and ease. Park Avenue is New York's grandest boulevard. It is stately and imposing. The brilliant yellow tulips in the spring and the lighted Christmas trees during the holidays make the avenue come alive to its many visitors and the few residents fortunate enough to call it home. The cachet of Park Avenue and the fine dining establishments, luxury hotels, and boutiques nearby have made the Upper East Side the most desirable and expensive neighborhood in New York.

Films and magazines depict the people who dwell on Park Avenue as though they have always lived there. And yet, only a small number of them actually grew up in this neighborhood. The majority of the avenue's residents are hard-working people who have put in the hours, made tremendous sacrifices, and stayed focused in order to be able to afford to live in this desirable location. If you don't believe me, take a walk along the avenue at six o'clock in the morning and you will see men and women leaving for work. These people understand that there are certain things that are *nonnegotiable* for success: formulating a plan, sticking with it for the long haul, and not giving up in the face of adversity.

The same is true of weight loss. We are constantly bombarded with advertisements for quick weight loss. But these messages are false and often dangerous. If all of these quick-fix diets were successful, why is the obesity epidemic reaching dangerously high levels in the United States? So, if you are hoping for a new quick-fix diet, then this is definitely *not* the book for you. But if you want to lose weight safely, and keep it off, then read on.

My name is Dr. Jana Klauer and my practice specializes in weight loss and nutrition. I attended the Mount Sinai School of Medicine in New York and completed my internship in Internal Medicine and residency in Rehabilitation Medicine at the Mount Sinai Hospital in New York. At the hospital, I treated a multitude of patients with the "diseases of civilization": high cholesterol, hypertension, diabetes, heart attack, and stroke. We have effective medicines that are able to control these conditions, but they do not cure them. Indeed, using medicine extends life, but the conditions remain. Most are directly attributable to an unhealthy diet and lack of physical exercise. Only when you take away the *cause* of the illness is health restored. I instructed my patients to lose weight, to visit a commercial weight-loss center. When they humored me and complied, the results were often suboptimal. They lost a few pounds, only to regain them. My patients were suffering with preventable illnesses. Because I cared deeply about their health, I knew that I must find a way to help them. But what more could I do? I needed more knowledge; I reasoned that, since my patients trusted me, if I advised them how to eat it might make a big difference. So I then obtained a master's degree in human nutrition from Columbia University, in a program specifically designed for clinicians.

After completing the program, I had the extraordinary privilege to manage a clinical trial with obese people at the New York Obesity Research Center at St. Luke's Roosevelt Hospital. In the trial I was able to expand my newfound competency in nutrition. I found the patients to be extraordinarily receptive; they actually enjoyed learning about nutrition, and lost weight! Additionally, having trained as a physical therapist prior to medical school, I am convinced of the positive effects that exercise can have on the body. So I encouraged them to begin an exercise program, and most agreed to this, also. I advised them to pick any form of exercise that they enjoyed and to do it daily. One gentleman who lived in Brooklyn and worked in lower Manhattan walked daily across the Brooklyn Bridge, to and from work. A nurse, on her lunch hour, walked daily with her colleagues in Central Park. A young law student ran along the Hudson River in the morning. Their choice of activity was as diverse as their occupations, but they all found a way to exercise consistently. To witness their success and their pride in achieving slimmer bodies was breathtaking. As they lost weight, medicines that had been taken for years were no longer necessary. They became healthy. Just as I had suspected, it was excessive weight that had caused illness.

Since 2000, my practice has been devoted entirely to nutrition and weight reduction. Because being physically active is an essential part of a healthy lifestyle, we have walking groups and all my patients are endlessly encouraged, needled, and cajoled to exercise. I often walk with them around the Central Park Reservoir. My office is located on Park Avenue and my patients are primarily highly successful business men and women, "ladies who lunch," and notable celebrities. They have enjoyed tremendous success due to their commitment to this lifestyle program. I invite you to do the same.

In this book, we will review the basics of diet and weight loss. Much of the information will be familiar, but I will explain the science of successful dieting so you know exactly what effect each and every food will have on your body. Once we have established the core "diet," we will discuss the *nonnegotiables*. They are amazingly simple and easily incorporated principles that you *must* add into your daily routine. They are called nonnegotiables because if you are serious about weight loss, YOU CANNOT SKIP THESE. They make all the difference in the world in helping my patients achieve their optimal weight. These are going to be your secret weapons as well.

Nonnegotiables

1. *Daily exercise.* You must schedule it into your routine. You need this for healthy muscles. If you don't exercise, you will get flabby and fat; it is that simple.
2. *Protein.* In a high-quality form, protein is vital for the functioning of your body. Include protein at every meal.
3. *Calcium.* This mineral is essential for increasing metabolism levels.

4. *Conquering your food cravings.* These can, and must, be managed. I will show you how to do this.
5. *Elimination of all processed food.* Processed food has no benefit to your health and also stimulates appetite.

These *nonnegotiable* principles will make all the difference between those who go on diets, lose weight, and regain it back, and those who get rid of excess pounds for good. I know you can do it, as I have seen my patients enjoy great results with this message. It is hard work, no doubt, but the results are enormously gratifying and, most important, lasting.

Here are the basics: My plan starts by getting your nutrition under control efficiently. At the foundation is a diet for weight loss and weight maintenance that is steeped in science. There are no fads, no gimmicks, no shortcuts or quick fixes. The diet is high in protein, omega-3 fats, and complex carbohydrates in the form of vegetables. This diet promotes not only faster weight reduction but a dramatic change in your overall health profile. You will learn how to eat foods that will keep you energized, satisfied, and looking your best. Even though my practice is located right next to many excellent Park Avenue plastic surgeons, I am not going to advocate liposuction, tummy tucks, or body lifts as a means to reduce weight. The first step requires your commitment to making those eating and lifestyle changes that will produce visible results.

I will make you a promise. If you give the plan two months, it will give you a slimmer, stronger, and healthier body. And you will look and feel ten years younger.

HOW THE RICH GET THIN

Chapter One

THE PARK AVENUE

MIND-SET

You can never be too rich or too thin.

—WALLIS SIMPSON, DUCHESS OF WINDSOR

•   •   •

The Upper East Side of Manhattan is one of the most exciting and dynamic places in the world. It is also one of the areas of highest concentrated wealth in the world. The people who live in the elegant apartments and town houses in our neighborhood have a lifestyle defined by long working hours, hectic schedules, and the pressure of always looking their best. They are under constant time constraint juggling work, deadlines, meetings and social obligations, domestic and international travel, plus personal commitments. Time is a very precious commodity in New York City, and not something to be wasted. Park Avenue people are constantly in a hurry to get to the next appointment, to conquer the next rung on the social ladder, and to achieve another professional success. They work hard, they play hard, and they demand the best of everything.

Men and women who have arrived at the pinnacle of success want to look and feel fabulous once they get there! Their occupations and social circles require that they "look the part." They strive not only to be chic; they want to be fashionably slim. But the excessive hours of working, high-profile entertaining, and abundance of the best foods also contribute to an expanding waistline. They don't plan for the midafternoon hunger by tossing a piece of fruit or a container of yogurt into their briefcase or Hermès bag, so by dinnertime they arrive at a restaurant famished and dive right into the bread basket; they postpone an exercise session until the end of the day instead of scheduling it for the first thing in the morning (a time when the session cannot be interrupted or forgotten); they cut their schedules too tight so that taxis are taken for distances that could easily be walked. In effect, it is an accumulation of time misspent that makes their weight gradually creep up.

For my patients to enjoy what they have worked so hard for, they must change their behavior and realize the truism that life and health are gifts. The magnificent mind and body that provided them with the good life can become old before its time if not treated with respect. By approaching eating and exercise with the same discipline that characterizes the rest of their lives, their excess weight is lost, and a vibrant, youthful appearance is regained.

What Is the Park Avenue Mind-Set?

People who can afford to live on Park Avenue (or in other upscale areas) exhibit certain recognizable character traits. Because residence in this prime area is so valued, these traits are also associated with financial success. They tend to be highly competitive, always in a hurry, impatient, status conscious, and they want to be noticed. They are often preoccupied with work. These traits are true for both males and females.

Women who are not working outside of the home and are married to successful men with the Park Avenue mind-set are often just as driven. These women often belong to charitable groups and raise millions of dollars for worthy causes they are passionate about. In fact, many organizations would not be able to exist without the tireless work of these dedicated women. However, there is an expectation that they have to look perfect at all times. There is an intense competitiveness to looking fabulous at this level.

Since the 1960s reign of such New York socialite icons as Slim

Keith, Doris Duke, and Babe Paley, dubbed the "beautiful people" by Diana Vreeland, the beloved editor of *Harper's Bazaar* and *Vogue*, the rich have been considered the great influencers of fashion, style, and culture. As Wallis Simpson, the American-born Duchess of Windsor, once said, "You can never be too rich or too thin." The Park Avenue princess lives, dresses, and dies by this motto. And she may unknowingly sacrifice her health to do so. While it may be true that you cannot really be too rich, you most definitely can be too thin. By maintaining a dangerously low weight to fit into sleek designer fashions, a woman may eliminate vital nutrition. The items that I find lacking most commonly in such people are dairy products and sufficient protein. In some cases, such extreme dieters are fighting a neverending battle with a body type they were born with, instead of eating sensibly to sustain the health of the body they have.

How Your Body Type Affects Weight Gain

Your body type is determined largely by genetics, over which we have no control. William Sheldon, M.D., first developed the concept that everyone is born with a certain body type. Dr. Sheldon outlined three basic body types: ectomorph, mesomorph, and endomorph.

- Ectomorph is the type that fashion magazines would have us aspire to: tall with long, thin limbs and little body fat. Most supermodels and basketball players are the ectomorph body type. It is an unrealistic goal for many people not born this type.
- Mesomorph body types are characterized by an athletic, strong, and compact body. The world's top figure skaters and tennis players tend to fall into the mesomorph category.
- Endomorphs are round and gain weight easily.

The body type that you were born with is the body type that you will have for life. It is one of your physical characteristics, just like your eye color. If your goal is to keep yourself in the best of health, by avoiding excess weight, exercising daily, and maintaining correct posture you will look fabulous *whatever* body type you possess.

BODY TYPES

Ectomorph—slim, lithe, long-limbed	Gisele Bundchen, Cindy Crawford, Chris Rock
Mesomorph—athletic body, muscular	Gabrielle Reece, Katie Couric, Sarah Jessica Parker, Mark Wahlberg, Andre Agassi, Kristi Yamaguchi
Endomorph—round, voluptuous	Queen Latifah, Danny DeVito, Roseanne, Dr. Ruth, Azzedine Alaia

Do You Need a Medicine Cabinet Makeover?

I have heard some pretty amazing stories from patients about the lengths they have gone to in order to lose weight: fad diets, smoking, laxatives, and even stimulants like amphetamines and cocaine. Losing weight by any of these methods can result in a disruption of the body's chemistry. While people may lose weight by such means, their health declines and they end up looking worse and worse.

Unscrupulous medical professionals, especially via the Internet, give ready access to a variety of dubious medications promising weight loss. Many of my patients have previously tried unsuccessfully to become thinner by taking such "miracle" pills and potions only to find that the drugs were sabotaging their health. Thyroid stimulants, diuretics, nervous system stimulants, and the like can take a strong mind and body and turn it into a medical emergency: Unnecessary thyroid medication will cause bone loss and arrhythmias. Diuretics are dehydrating and put a strain on the heart. Stimulants cause an increase in both blood pressure and heart rate. Yet I have seen many patients who, out of desperation, have resorted to these means.

Don't become lured by an unhealthy solution to excess weight. There is no place in your life for this!

Drugs That Cause Weight Gain

A number of prescription and over-the-counter medications are associated with significant weight gain. Unfortunately, patients are not always told in advance about this unwelcome side effect: A weight gain occurs and the patient doesn't know why.

These medications are frequent causes of weight gain:

- *Antidepressants:* Fluoxetine (Prozac), sertraline (Zoloft), and paroxetine (Paxil) are effective antidepressants but can increase weight. A different class of antidepressant also associated with weight gain is mirtazapine (Remeron). For someone who is depressed, these drugs can lift the heavy emotional load; however, they should only be prescribed by a competent psychiatrist—*never* purchase them on the Internet. Antidepressants that do *not* increase weight are bupropion (Wellbutrin) and nefazodone (Serzone).
- *Antipsychotics*
- *Antiseizure medications*: Just about all of these medications cause some weight gain with the exception of topiramate (Topamax), which may cause weight loss.
- *Oral contraceptives* (Yasmin may cause weight loss)
- *Corticosteroids* (for asthma, autoimmune conditions, and allergies)
- *Antihistamines* (for allergies)
- *Beta blockers* (for high blood pressure)

If you are taking any of the above drugs and have gained weight, do not assume that your doctor knows that you are experiencing weight gain, because it does not occur in all patients. Discuss your weight change with your physician. There are alternative medications that may work just as well for you. For example, decongestants may be substituted for antihistamines; ACE inhibitors or calcium channel blockers may be substituted for beta blockers; antidepressants that do not cause weight gain as a side effect can be substituted for those that promote weight gain; barrier methods can replace oral contraceptives.

Julia is a thirty-eight-year-old mother of twins who experienced a depression after the end of her ten-year marriage. She consulted a psychiatrist, and was treated with psychotherapy and a high dosage of paroxetine (Paxil). After several months, her depression resolved and she stopped seeing her psychiatrist. But four years and thirty pounds later, this young woman was still taking the medication plus an oral contraceptive and an antihistamine. Distressed because her own weight-loss efforts were not working, she sought my help to lose weight.

When I spoke with Julia, she was amazed to hear of the combined effects of her medications, as their potential for weight gain had never been explained to her. First, I suggested that she consult with her psychiatrist, whom she had not seen in over three years, to assess whether she could safely eliminate the antidepressant; she had been obtaining paroxetine (Paxil) prescriptions from her primary care physician. Her psychiatrist agreed that she did not need the medicine anymore. She was able to reduce her antihistamine, which she took for hay fever, to a minimal amount on high-pollen days. Julia lost the excess thirty pounds in about three months. She is now happy, confident, and slimmer.

The drugs were probably appropriate at the time they were prescribed, but she should have been told that weight gain was a possibility. Also, her use of medications had continued for longer than necessary. Additionally, mixing medications had had a cumulative effect with regard to weight gain.

The Myths of Diet Drugs

Baby boomers are known to demand the "instant gratification" factor. This is a real problem with weight management because there are no shortcuts. A magic pill that will cut appetite, raise metabolism, and give you a supermodel body does not exist. There are medications that treat obesity, but they only work when combined with diet and exercise. One of the worst things that a physician can do is to prescribe any of these medications without explaining the limitations of the drug, and not stressing that they won't work without changing the diet. And, like every medicine, they all have side effects.

Drugs That Reduce Food Intake

The drugs listed are prescription medications and should only be taken under a doctor's supervision. The Internet has made these medications available online, which has resulted in serious medical consequences, including death. If you have a significant amount of weight to lose, consult with your doctor about a diet and exercise plan.

Phentermine, which decreases appetite, is the most widely prescribed and oldest prescription weight-loss medication, having been around for thirty years. It stimulates the release of norepinephrine and dopamine from nerve terminals. As such, it increases the heart rate and raises blood pressure. Other side effects are dry mouth, constipation, and insomnia. Because of its effect on blood pressure and the heart rate, usage of phentermine should be carefully monitored, and the suggested treatment period is no longer than six weeks.

Several years ago, the combination of phentermine and fenfluramine (Phen Fen) was thought to be the answer for quick and easy weight loss. People who took the drug experienced dramatic reduction in weight and felt almost no hunger. But soon this "miracle drug" was found to be responsible for damage to the heart valves. Tragically, several deaths resulted from the drug and it has now been removed from the market. The gold standard of weight loss has always been a healthy diet and exercise. Don't risk your life by using this dangerous drug combination.

Sibutramine (Meridia) is a norepinephrine and serotonin reuptake inhibitor. Weight loss is dose dependent: It affects the appetite center of the brain, where it increases satiety so you feel full faster and with a smaller quantity of food. The drug has been extremely well studied. Clinical studies have shown that sibutramine is effective and safe, if properly prescribed. Blood pressure and heart rate must be monitored, however, as sibutramine can cause a dangerous rise in blood pressure. Sibutramine should never be used in patients with a history of coronary artery disease, congestive heart failure, cardiac arrhythmia, or stroke. Because its action affects the brain, it is not safe to take with most antidepressant drugs. The side effects of sibutramine include dry mouth, constipation, and insomnia.

Orlistat (Xenical) is unique in that it does not enter the circulation but rather works in the digestive system to block the absorption of fat, which is then eliminated from the body through the stool. If you eat too much fat, diarrhea is the unhappy result. Orlistat works well because its action is entirely within the digestive tract; it doesn't interact with other medications, and does not raise blood pressure or the heart rate. However, because it blocks absorption of fat, it blocks the absorption of the fat-soluble vitamins, and these should be taken separately.

The truth is that there is no ideal weight-loss pill. Medications are suitable for some people, and can assist in raising the metabolism forward, but they are useless if exercise and an optimal diet are not in place. You won't need drugs with my plan.

Nonprescription Weight-Loss Drugs

Drugs that are sold over the counter and over the Internet promise weight loss but deliver little in the way of results. Weight-loss supplements fall into two basic categories: those that claim to suppress appetite and those that block the absorption of food. The appetite suppressors contain caffeinelike substances (such as ephedra or ma huang, which is now banned). Studies in animals have indicated a small appetite-suppressant effect, but the human studies have been too brief to support the claims.

Appetite suppressants have the side effects of increasing blood pressure, headache, insomnia, and heart palpitations. You will feel jittery, as is the case with too much coffee. The absorption-blockers seem to have a small effect, but cause side effects of bloating and gastrointestinal complaints.

The bottom line is: Over-the-counter and Internet-sold drugs do not work, and are usually not safe. Save your money. You have to change your diet and exercise routine to see a meaningful change in your weight.

THE PARK AVENUE MYSTIQUE

According to the New York City Department of Parks and Recreation, what is now Park Avenue was originally laid out in the 1811 Commissioners' Plan as Fourth Avenue. In 1832, the long, narrow strip down the middle of the island was granted to the New York and Harlem Railroad, which ran horse-drawn cars along its path, starting with a run between Union Square and Twenty-third Street. By 1834, the service operated from Prince Street to the Upper East Side. Though given its present name in 1888, it was the 1903 conversion from steam to electric train power and the 1913 completion of the present Grand Central Terminal that paved the way for Park Avenue's future. The previously open rail yards and tracks north of the terminal were covered over between 1921 and 1924, and the avenue's wide, landscaped center medians gave credibility to its name. Subsequently, the wide malls were narrowed to their present configuration, to accommodate wider traffic lanes.

Today Park Avenue consists of rows of apartment buildings on the east and west sides of the street, separated in the center of the avenue by wide, planted islands. As the seasons change, so do the lovely gardens. In summer, the plantings consist of begonias; spring, tulips and flowering apple blossoms; fall, chrysanthemums; and the end of the year brings festive and beautifully lighted Christmas trees. The apartment buildings lining Park Avenue embody conservative elegance. Some of the grandest residences were constructed between 1920 and 1930 by Rosario Candela, with only one apartment per floor. Candela's apartments created the "off the foyer" layout, in which the foyer was an additional room that set the tone for the entry into the formal living space. Candela's well-constructed apartments had thick walls, large rooms with elegant double moldings, and very high ceilings. Born in Palermo, Italy, Rosario Candela's father was a plasterer. The architect Candela's own story represents fulfillment of the American dream, because today his elegant buildings are landmark structures and epitomize New York City living at the highest level. Our office is located in one of the beautiful buildings built by Rosario Candela.

DO YOU HAVE THE PARK AVENUE MIND-SET?

1. Do you have a sense of time urgency? Are you always in a rush?
2. Do you inhale your food—are you always the first one at the table to finish a meal?
3. Do you talk so fast that people tell you to slow down?
4. Will you sacrifice a health-promoting behavior, such as a yoga class, for an extra hour at the office or to take on one more afterschool activity for your children?
5. Do you reach for a cookie or candy bar to power yourself through the afternoon?
6. Do you speed up at the yellow light?
7. Would you rather spend time working than working out?
8. Do you find yourself falling into bed at night and saying, "Not tonight, dear," because you have no energy left for sex?
9. Do you talk on your cell phone or eat meals while driving?
10. Do you eat on the run; i.e., in the car, at the airport?
11. Do you frequently order in or order room service?
12. Do you hit the mini bar the minute you check into your hotel room?
13. Are your thumbs sore from using your Blackberry all day long?
14. Are you a multitasker?
15. Are you addicted to caffeine?

If you answered yes to two or more of these questions, you *need* my plan. And the more affirmative answers you gave, then the more likely the plan will be successful for you, because of your drive. The positive aspects of these traits focus you on your work; the negative aspects cause you to neglect your health.

Since knowledge is power, I suggest that you use this behavior pattern to improve your health and to identify what you are doing wrong. Your strong determination can actually be an asset in correcting the negative health patterns. When these people see that something is broken, they fix it!

How the Park Avenue Mind-Set Could Work for You

Sandra is a forty-five-year-old single woman who is a senior portfolio manager at an investment bank. Since becoming a senior executive, Sandra had allowed her weight to gradually creep upward, due to long hours at the office, little or no time for exercise, and eating out frequently, choosing rich foods. Sandra camouflaged her extra weight with expensive couture suits. While her overall health was good, her total cholesterol was just over 250 mg/dl. Her waistline had increased to 37 inches. Both of these are independent risk factors for disease. Sandra was accustomed to being "in charge" and informed me that she "knew all about eating and how to lose weight," but clearly she needed help with this. Sandra's work required her to entertain clients for dinner five nights of the week. Her business dinners were usually at four-star restaurants and always included fine wines. Sandra had an active social life that also included alcohol. If an average drink accounts for 200 kcal—then Sandra was consuming about 4,000 kcal per week just in the form of alcohol! One pound is equivalent to 3,500 kcal—so theoretically just by eliminating alcohol it would be possible for her to lose approximately one pound per week.

These are the changes I suggested for Sandra:

1. Eliminate alcohol. Drink only mineral water at business dinners. Initially, like all of my patients, she resisted this idea but, once she agreed to it, she was amazed at how easy it was. She ordered a large bottle of San Pellegrino and lime slices for the table. Her clients did not seem to mind her abstinence, and she also became more efficient at these meetings.

2. Stay away from the bread basket and order a crudités platter to be served prior to dinner. Sandra saved calories by eliminating simple carbohydrates and was a big hit with her clients. They loved the elegantly presented, chilled vegetables and thought this was a gracious gesture by their hostess. (After all, they were trying to control their weight, too!)

3. Order two appetizers as your dinner or cut the main course in half. Restaurant portions are just too big.

4. Make daily aerobic exercise a priority. No more excuses!

Because Sandra enjoyed being in control and saw the program was working for her, she focused her energy on this. After six months, Sandra had lost 35 pounds and normalized her cholesterol. She realized that simply being in a fancy restaurant is not a green light for passively overeating but rather another opportunity to control a situation. I was able to make her Park Avenue mind-set work to her advantage!

Jackie is one of my favorite success stories, and her story was actually published in *Modern Bride* because it was so inspiring to other women. Exactly one year before she was due to wed her high school sweetheart, Jackie resolved to lose 25 pounds. At five foot six, the bride-to-be was concerned about the weight she had put on in her twenties, a decade she spent drinking and partying. She needed a jumpstart to get her going. When I first inquired about her eating habits, Jackie told me that she only had coffee in the morning. As I probed the nature of this beverage, I learned that she was starting her day with a Starbucks Caffè Mocha Grande with whipped cream. We looked this up and she was astounded to find that the calorie content was a whopping 660 calories! Jackie switched to Skim Cappuccino Grande. As she waited in line at the local Starbucks, she warned her fellow caffeine lovers about the calorie content of her former favorite "coffee" beverage. I put Jackie on a regimen of running, weight training, and a healthier diet. She restructured her eating habits by reading nutritional labels; eating half portions when dining out; and substituting fruits, vegetables, proteins, and whole grains for sweets and fast foods. She cut down on her alcohol intake by switching to occasional low-calorie wine spritzers. As a result, the newly trim bride had her wedding dress taken in from a size 10 to a 6, and marched down the aisle like a diva!

Here is another typical patient of mine—John, a fifty-six-year-old attorney who heads a law firm representing the music industry. His demanding schedule calls for almost weekly trips to the West Coast. His long workdays and extensive travel resulted in his becoming 75 pounds overweight—and exhausted. When he finally saw his internist, John was diagnosed with high cholesterol, high blood pressure, and type

2 diabetes mellitus. John's lifestyle had made him wealthy in a material sense but had bankrupted his health! Luckily, his internist referred John to me. John, a highly motivated individual, was resolved to change his life for the better. He readily implemented the diet and exercise recommendations that I made. Travel was a particular concern. Although John always flew first class, he realized that the food served by the airline was not what he should eat while trying to lose weight. He followed my suggestion and took an 8-ounce container of plain low-fat yogurt, cut-up vegetables, and low-fat string cheese with him on flights. He drank only water while on board the plane. While in Los Angeles, he always stayed at the Peninsula in Beverly Hills. He asked his hotel to pack a lunch of smoked salmon and vegetables for the return flight. John made a point of walking two miles daily on his home treadmill and on business trips. As his weight came down, John was able to jog comfortably.

Over time, as his cholesterol, blood pressure, and diabetes resolved, I was able to reduce and subsequently discontinue all of John's medications. He made his health a priority and did not come up with excuses to avoid living a health-promoting lifestyle. He simply followed the Klauer Plan one day at a time. While continuing to manage the responsibilities and pressures of a demanding career, he chose to also reverse the illness within his body. He changed his life. He was still under the same time pressure but now made time for his health.

I tell Sandra's, Jackie's, and John's stories because: (a) If they were able to make these changes, then so can you; and (b) by committing to my diet and exercise plan, you can improve your health. When you consider each change that these very different people made, you realize that these are things that anyone can do. Their strong will and determination to persist are what enabled these people to change their lives. They did not give up and they did not give in! Day after day, they followed the plan that they saw was working until they reached their targets.

The key is to keep your goal in sight. It is your health and well-being that are at stake, and these are high stakes, indeed. Treat a weight-loss plan like a business plan—have a goal and take the necessary steps to get there. As another successful patient stated, you must "plan the work and work the plan!" It will not happen overnight but if you persist, you will get there. The wonderful news is that when you follow this plan you can expect to look and feel better than you have in years.

Chapter Two

PROTEIN — THE ANCHOR

OF YOUR DIET

*Get health. No labor, effort, nor exercise
that can gain it must be grudged.*

—RALPH WALDO EMERSON

•   •   •

Build and Repair

At the cornerstone of my program lies the concept of "build and repair."
While there is a continuous healthy debate as to what constitutes the
best diet for weight loss, there are several facts that cannot be ignored.
These have been shown to be true through clinical trials and can benefit
the individual who wants to be slim and healthy.

Indisputable Diet Gems

1. Weight loss occurs more rapidly with a high-protein diet.
2. Eating starchy carbohydrates, such as cookies, bread, and pasta,
    allows hunger to return more quickly than if protein is eaten.
3. Vegetables and fruit are all-natural sources of vitamins, miner-
    als, and antioxidants, plus they are filling.

Based on these hard and fast facts, it should appear obvious that to lose excess weight you should consume more protein and more vegetables and limited fruit, while eliminating starchy and sugary carbohydrates. (I suggest that you limit fruit to 2 servings per day while attempting to lose weight, due to the higher calorie content.)

Science has long demonstrated that added sugars have little dietary value, serving primarily as sweeteners and bulking agents, and as sources of unnecessary calories. For example, a study published in *The Journal of the American Medical Association* in August 2004 showed that a higher consumption of sugar-sweetened beverages is associated with greater weight gain and an increased risk for developing type 2 diabetes in women.[1] In fact, according to the United States Department of Agriculture (USDA), the average American consumes 158 pounds of various sugars annually.

The core concept is to build and repair. Protein provides the building blocks for the body. All tissues that are growing or rebuilding require protein. Our bodies are in a constant state of renewal. We require protein to synthesize hormones and enzymes, and to repair and rebuild muscles and our organs. If we are actively exercising, we require more protein than if we are inactive, because protein is necessary for maintenance of the muscles.

The amount of protein that we need is around 1 gram per kilogram of body weight per day for a sedentary person. Since you are going to be more active, you should strive for a little bit more than that. For example, a 120-pound female needs 60 to 70 g (a little over 2 ounces) of protein; a 170-pound male needs 80 to 90 g (about 3 ounces) of protein.

An interesting fact about protein is that it is three times more expensive for your body to metabolize than carbohydrates. You actually need three times more calories to digest protein than to digest carbohydrates or fats.[2] While carbohydrates give you an immediate boost in energy, due to their faster assimilation, proteins become incorporated into your body through multiple steps and each step requires calories.

High-quality proteins are: egg whites, any seafood—including shellfish—organic dairy products, organic poultry, and organic meat. I did not include plant protein in the list because, with the exception of soy protein plants lack essential amino acids. You need to consume amino acids that exist only in living animals.

Low blood glucose signals hunger. Most people reach for a starchy or sugary carbohydrate snack when they are hungry, because these snacks cause the blood glucose to rise rapidly. Unfortunately, the type of carbohydrate most people consume is in the form of processed food with little nutrition. These empty-calorie carbohydrate snacks fill supermarket shelves. Sure, you get an energy boost, but it doesn't last, and soon you are hungry again. Do these snacks help you to "build and repair"? The answer is a resounding NO WAY! Processed carbohydrate snacks are unsatisfying and will make you fat.

Items that masquerade as protein bars are not examples of high-quality protein. They are processed and unnatural snacks. The protein contained within the bar is manufactured from various amino acids, held together with a gumlike substance and made palatable with artificial flavorings and, often, lots of sugar. For example, a chocolate–peanut butter PowerBar Performance Bar is packed with 20 g of sugars, which is twice the amount of sugar you get in a single Krispy Kreme Original Glazed Doughnut! A power bar sounds like a good idea because of all the added vitamins, but all that sugar cancels out its health benefits. Even power bars sold at health food stores are heavily sweetened with honey or fructose. The best nutrition comes from pure, whole foods. Next time you seek an energy boost from a sweetened processed food, think again. Overconsumption of added sugars is a significant contributor to the obesity epidemic in America, and can tip you into type 2 diabetes.

Protein Quality

The type of protein consumed is also important. The quality of a protein is determined by how much of the protein is available to the body, whether it contains essential amino acids, and the quantity and quality of the associated fat. Protein is composed of subunits called "amino acids." In all of nature there are twenty-one kinds of amino acids. Each type of protein is dependent upon the arrangement of its amino acids, much the way a word is composed of a unique arrangement of only some of the twenty-six letters of the alphabet. Protein quality is determined by whether all the amino acids that the body requires are present. Another factor of quality is the amount and type of fat in the food.

Protein and fat are like Siamese twins: They are always together.

The gold standard against which we measure all protein is the white of an egg. The egg white is the most concentrated form of protein because its associated fat is contained within the yolk. Because the yolk can be separated from the white, the fat content can easily be avoided. No fat is present in the white of an egg. Egg whites contain all the essential amino acids, and the white is pure protein. Egg whites offer the convenience of what I consider a healthy fast food. You can crack open a few eggs, separate them, add some sliced vegetables, and whip up a delicious low-fat egg-white omelet in minutes.

The next best sources of protein in terms of quality are fish and low-fat dairy products. Fish and dairy contain all the essential amino acids. The fat present in fish is omega-3 fat, which is anti-inflammatory and cardio-protective. Eating fat-free dairy products is a healthy way to obtain protein.

Next in the protein hierarchy are poultry and lean meat. Meat contains the essential amino acids but has saturated fat. Poultry also contains saturated fat, but it is found mainly in the skin.

Last come vegetables, grains, and legumes. They don't have all the essential amino acids and while they contain omega-3 fats, they are part carbohydrate, which dilutes the protein. Vegetables, grains, and legumes are terrific foods for us, but their protein quality is not as good as that of other sources. You need to eat them in combination, and eat a lot more of them to obtain the level of amino acids found in animal sources of protein.

Another key aspect of the Park Avenue mind-set is the art of enjoying life to its fullest. If you fill your days with little pleasures, the sum total of your life will be that much more enriched. For example, if you are going to eat seafood, make it the finest quality you can find. Instead of having lumpfish from a tin, treat yourself to the 20-gram presentation of Caviar Tsar Imperial Beluga from Petrossian and savor every last morsel. Everything you put into your mouth should be a sensual experience. Eat slowly instead of gobbling down your food, so you can taste each bite. Eat less, but eat well!

Your ultimate goal is to maximize the highest-quality protein to build and repair.

Much has been written about the poor eating habits in the United States, and a great deal of blame has been placed upon our overconsumption of cheap fast food. While it may be true for the majority of the country, it is also true that wealthy people, who can afford the best food, do not always choose it. The cause for this is primarily a lack of basic knowledge. No matter how intelligent and well educated people are, it is surprising how little they know about nutrition. They can tell you everything that you want to know about the bestseller list, the intricacies of world history and politics, the great art of the world, and so on, and yet, when it comes to understanding basic information about the food that they and their families consume—they may be virtually ignorant.

Whether you actually live on Park Avenue or simply aspire to such a lifestyle, it is your responsibility to choose the best foods for your optimum health. And that includes consuming, wherever possible, organic sources of protein, even though organic foods generally cost a little more.

Grass-Fed Meat

While the majority of meat in the United States is grain fed and hormone enhanced, it is best to choose meat that is raised in a natural manner. Grass-fed beef comes from animals that are allowed to graze in pastures, not crowded into large-scale feedlots and given a corn-heavy diet.

Why is that important? The animal's diet affects the type of fat present in the meat. The meat is lower in fat and contains a higher percentage of omega-3 fat. It is free of hormones and antibiotics, substances that the American Medical Association has publicly opposed because of a potential link to antibiotic resistance. Therefore, it makes more sense to consume meat from animals that grow and mature naturally. However, the grain of the meat has a more robust, heartier texture and may take some time to get used to. If you find this meat too grainy for your tastes, seek out other farmers who do not exclusively feed their cows grass, but allow some grain, and avoid antibiotics and hormones. Their meat may have a softer texture.

> While researching grass-fed beef sources, I looked for New York City restaurants that served organic beef. I came across Beppe, a terrific Italian place in the Flatiron District. Their menu consists of dishes prepared with organic ingredients grown on their Tutto Bene farm in upstate New York. I visited the restaurant myself to determine whether it suited my diet, so I could recommend it to my patients. I started with the Pontormo salad, which is a warm salad of field greens with a tarragon vinaigrette made with fresh tarragon from the farm, and accompanied by scrambled organic eggs. To follow, I tried the roasted quail that was served on beans with rosemary, which is not something I would normally order. It was wonderful. Quail is a wild bird, and because it is wild, it does not have as much fat as chicken and there is more dark meat.

To help you locate the best-quality meats, I have prepared a useful selection of Web addresses (see Resources).

> To build and repair with the best materials requires keeping saturated fat low and including omega-3 fats.
>
> Plant proteins are incomplete, meaning they do not supply all the essential amino acids. But, on the positive side, plants supply omega-3 fat and fiber. We require 25 to 35 g of fiber daily. So you can eat your beans, but make sure that you include higher-quality proteins as well. Beans, although high in protein, are also a source of starchy carbohydrates. There are many wonderful varieties, including black-eyed peas, fava beans, and cannellini, but these should be eaten in moderation.
>
> *(continued)*

PROTEIN SCORECARD

FOOD	PROTEIN QUALITY	ASSOCIATED FAT	GRAMS
Egg whites	Excellent	None	7 g per egg
Fish	Excellent	Omega-3 fat	7 g per ounce
Skim milk	Excellent	None	10 g per cup
Yogurt	Excellent	None if from skim milk	15 g per 8-ounce cup
Poultry	Excellent	Sat. fat, mostly in skin	7 g per ounce
Meat	Excellent	Sat. fat	7 g per ounce
Beans	Fair	Omega-3 fat	7 g per ½ cup dried (cooked)

Be resourceful in obtaining the best choices for your body. I attended a benefit dinner recently in a beautiful Upper East Side town house for the charity "Save Venice." Prime rib of beef was the main course. That was it—no other choices. As the waiter came to inquire how I would like my beef cooked, I asked him if I could have fish instead. The hunk of rare beef just appeared in front of all the guests alongside potatoes au gratin and some haricots verts that were swimming in a buttery sauce. The waiter brought me a gorgeous halibut steak dressed with chopped olives and tomatoes and other fresh vegetables. I was seated between two men who were served the beef and they both said, in unison, "We should have had that." The moral of the story is that you should not be afraid to ask the kitchen to accommodate your special requests. If you are invited to a gala or a wedding party, you may even request a healthy meal in advance, as you can do on overseas flights. Or ask for an entrée-size portion of a healthy appetizer. Vegetarian, fish, or even chicken may easily be substituted for less-healthy beef dishes or pasta. Speak up, you will be surprised at how easy it is!

Pre-Illness Conditions

When I meet patients in my reception area for the first time, they are often expensively dressed and talking on their cell phones (they don't want to waste a minute). After I usher them into my consultation room and take their comprehensive medical history, I often find that they are taking medications for elevated blood pressure, high cholesterol, coronary disease, and anxiety. They know that they need to lose weight. Their blood work may show that they have signs of prediabetes. Once inside the examination room, when the expensive clothes are set aside, the seriousness of their condition truly becomes evident. Thinning hair, premature wrinkling of the skin, poor posture, and inadequate muscle mass are evidence of poor lifestyle choices. Although the scars from liposuction may be evident, their waist size is often increased. Liposuction can remove only subcutaneous fat—it cannot touch the dangerous visceral fat, which is deeper.

> *Waistline Wisdom: A waist measuring greater than 35 inches for a female or greater than 40 inches for a male is an indication of visceral fat, which is considered to increase the risk for diabetes and is part of the constellation of symptoms that define the metabolic syndrome.*

"Visceral fat" refers to fat beneath the abdominal muscle layer. This is a very dangerous type of fat that predisposes an individual to diabetes, many types of cancer, and cardiovascular disease. This fat is inaccessible to liposuction. Although these people are not sick clinically, they are not really well, either. They are in a state of "pre-illness." Allowed to progress, the pre-illness phase will develop into debilitating illness.

Pre-illness should serve as a wake-up call to take action with respect to health. Unfortunately, it is also true that most people are unaware that they are in peril. They think that by taking a pill they have cured their high blood pressure and high cholesterol. Although the drugs that we have today are invaluable and have extended many lives, they are not the true solution to the problem. This is similar to thinking that by coloring your hair, you will no longer have gray hair. Just wait a few weeks and the roots will show again. The same is true with medications—your cholesterol may be controlled with these but, once you stop taking them, watch your numbers shoot back up!

Review the following "pre-illness" characteristics and honestly assess if any of these apply to you.

1. Has your waistline grown? Do you feel that you are accumulating extra pounds around the middle?
2. Is your cholesterol too high? Do you take medication to control it?
3. Is your blood pressure too high? Do you take medication to control it?
4. Do you have trouble sleeping?
5. Do you exercise regularly?
6. Are you depressed?
7. Have you gained more than 10 pounds within the last year?
8. When was the last time you had sex?

Reversal of the pre-illness phase takes more than pills, it requires an aggressive commitment to changing the unhealthy behaviors that created the problem.

High Cholesterol

Although there are strong genetic factors in cholesterol metabolism, lifestyle factors are the dominant players. While it is true that we inherit a predisposition toward a certain cholesterol level, our choices in food and lifestyle are the keys in keeping this in a healthy range. The types of foods we eat greatly influence if our cholesterol is high or low. Studies of populations with low risk for heart disease and low cholesterol levels show diets high in vegetables and fruits and low in saturated fat. Eating a diet high in processed food and high in saturated fat, with excess calories, is perhaps the worst thing that we can do for our cholesterol and heart. But this is what most people do, and they rationalize this by telling themselves that their cholesterol is fine because of the medication they take to keep the level down. This is just not so! A diet with high amounts of fruits, vegetables, and fish, with fat in the form of olive oil and nuts, can actually lower the cholesterol without the use of medication. It is delicious, and populations with a low risk for cardiovascular disease already eat in this fashion.

Here is an adjunct to a healthy diet: Try adding ginger juice. Ginger has long been recognized as a natural digestive aid and its flavor kick enhances almost any type of food. It is terrific for cooking and for marinating fish, vegetables, and chicken, and you can even make a festive spritzer out of it by mixing it with sparkling water. Visit www.gingerpeople.com for more information.

NOT ALL FISH ARE ALIKE

Every 29 seconds, someone in the United States suffers a heart attack. If you are trying to eat more fish for a healthy heart, keep in mind that only fish that is broiled, grilled, or baked actually protects against heart disease. The American Heart Association recommends two or more weekly servings. The best kinds of fish to eat are those high in omega-3 fatty acids, such as salmon, halibut, bluefish, and red snapper. Omega-3 fats are thought to increase the so-called good HDL cholesterol and lower triglycerides.

(continued)

Here's a great protein find. Ed's Kasilof Seafoods is an Alaskan fishery where the salmon is wild, not farmed. The waters of Alaska are not as high in mercury as the Atlantic Ocean. They feature canned salmon that comes in 7.5-ounce cans—good for two nice portions at 120 calories per portion, 17 g of protein, 0 carbs, and rich in omega-3 fats. They also carry canned, smoked, flaked salmon that is delicious, and other varieties of seafoods, including halibut and king crab. Call 1-800-982-2377 or visit their Web site, www.kasilofseafoods.com.

Inflammation

Visceral fat causes a state of chronic inflammation. Chronic inflammation is harmful to the body, particularly affecting the coronary arteries. We are able to determine if inflammation is present through a laboratory test for high-sensitivity C-reactive protein, or CRP. High-sensitivity CRP tells us if the arteries to the heart are inflamed. It has long been known that about 50 percent of individuals having a heart attack test for normal cholesterol levels. Cholesterol alone doesn't tell the whole story. Recent studies have proven that the presence of chronic inflammation—a high CRP level—is just as important a risk for having a heart attack as is high cholesterol. If *both* cholesterol and CRP are elevated, the risk is quadrupled.

Chronic inflammation is caused by excessive weight. For years it was assumed that fat cells were simply storage cells. We could not have been more wrong! The fat cell is an extremely active cell, metabolically. It produces hormones that are sensed in the brain, and proteins that signal other cells and cause a chronic inflammatory state in the body. Because of this wide range of actions, the fat cells are now recognized as the largest endocrine organ in the body. Excessive fat, by its inflammatory effect, can be as deadly as a bullet to your heart. It is excessive fat that causes a high level of CRP. Losing weight causes a *measurable* reduction in this inflammation, reflected by lower blood levels of CRP. Think about it: Just by losing weight, you can rid yourself of inflammatory proteins that could give you a heart attack.

Blood Pressure

Blood pressure, too, is strongly affected by lifestyle factors. Everyone knows that stress increases blood pressure, but not everyone is aware of the very impressive studies that have shown a diet high in fruits, vegetables, and dairy products can improve blood pressure. By adding calcium to our diet, we can lower blood pressure! Include exercise, and it will go down even more. Lose weight, and it will become normal. As a physician, I have witnessed this fact time and time again in my own patients.

Belly Fat

As they gain weight, men find that their waist size increases and they must purchase new, larger belts and pants. An increase in waist size is not only unsightly but unhealthy. Belly fat is a risk for cardiovascular disease. If you are male and your waist size is greater than your chest size, you could be on the road to heart problems.

An increase in abdominal fat is especially troubling for middle-aged women. The reasons for fat deposition in this area are related to estrogen status. Before puberty, a young girl and boy have the same silhouettes. At puberty, estrogen causes fat to be preferentially distributed on girls' hips and thighs, giving the characteristic female shape. This is believed to be an evolutionary trait that enabled a woman to carry a child to term in times of famine. As a woman enters midlife, and estrogen production declines, fat is deposited around the waist. While she may have had a slim waist as a young woman, now it can seem as if every additional pound is deposited around her middle. This is dangerous fat, as I have mentioned, and predisposes women to cardiovascular disease. After menopause, a woman's risk for a heart attack approaches that of a man; and women don't do as well after a heart attack as men. Excessive calories put this fat belt on, but you can get rid of it by eating right and committing to regular aerobic exercise. A recent study of overweight women showed that just by walking briskly for 45 minutes daily, women were able to decrease their waist size by 3 inches. A 3-inch weight loss around the midsection can translate to dropping a size in pants or skirts—or letting you get into your favorite jeans again without lying on your bed and holding your breath.

Did you know that 8 pounds usually equals one dress size?

Snoring

As weight is gained during the pre-illness phase, men may notice that their shirt collars are becoming too tight. Fat deposited here not only results in sagging jowls but also in snoring. A neck size greater than 17 inches is the danger mark. The fatty deposits around the neck compress the breathing structures while reclining and, as the muscles become relaxed during sleep, snoring develops. This can become a real problem between spouses, causing marital strife and daytime sleepiness for husband and wife. Alcohol makes snoring worse. A condition known as *sleep apnea* can develop; in this case breathing stops, causing the individual to awaken to regain breath. This can result in chronic daytime exhaustion.

Interestingly, although my patients have the financial means to avail themselves of the best foods, they often do not know what these foods are. Although they have indulged in some of the top medical spas in the country, they are still troubled with disease that is almost entirely preventable. The fast-paced and privileged lifestyle led by many of my patients does not include the basic tools to live long and healthily.

Harold is a sixty-two-year-old partner in one of the major financial investment banks in New York City. He was forced to see me by his wife of thirty years, Joan. She is a superachiever in her own right. Besides successfully raising three children, she has chaired major philanthropic organizations and benefit committees. But Joan, elegant and energetic, does more than just give money to these organizations; she also works in soup kitchens and tutors underprivileged children. Raised by a single mother because her father had died at age thirty-five from a massive heart attack, Joan inherited a predisposition for an un-

(continued)

healthy cholesterol level from her father, but has done everything in her power to stay in good health. She exercises daily, doesn't smoke, and has maintained her size 4 figure throughout her marriage. Harold, on the other hand, is a different story. Although he does not have a hereditary predisposition for cardiovascular disease, he had not taken care of his health. His weight ballooned to over 300 pounds and his waist size was 54 inches. He ate at the finest restaurants and he did not deprive himself of anything. He belonged to a number of prestigious country clubs; golf was his only form of exercise (even though he had a full gym in his home that was used only by his wife). His stress level at work was off the charts. Harold's laboratory work showed that his total cholesterol was over 300 mg/dl (normal is less than 200) and his CRP was 5.1 (normal is less than 0.8).

Clearly, Harold needed help. Joan was terrified that she would lose her husband to heart disease just as she had lost her father. And in fact, not only was Harold's risk for cardiovascular disease high, but his weight also increased his risk for cancer. Harold personified the pre-illness phase. Because of his devotion to his extraordinary wife, he agreed to follow my recommendations.

I gave Harold the diet plan that is outlined in this book and he followed it to the letter. He often told me how surprisingly easy it was for him to follow the plan and marveled at his lack of hunger. For exercise, he took morning walks in Central Park with Joan, who keeps up a brisk pace. Later he hired a personal trainer. Over the course of one year, Harold lost 100 pounds, and 16 inches from his waist. Harold looks and feels like a younger man and his wife is delighted with his new energy. Harold did not come into this world with risk factors for disease, as his wife did. Harold created these risk factors with poor food choices and lack of physical exercise. But he was able to turn this around by diet and exercise. His cholesterol and CRP are now normal. Harold lost his risk factors, and so can you.

ARE YOU IN THE PRE-ILLNESS PHASE?

1. Is your blood pressure above 120/80?
2. Is your LDL cholesterol above 100 mg/dl?
3. Is your HDL cholesterol under 55 if you are a male or under 65 if you are a female?
4. Is your fasting blood sugar over 100?
5. Is your waist size greater than 35 inches if you are a female, or 40 inches if you are a male? Are you buying larger belts?
6. Are you overweight? Do you wear more than two sizes larger than you did when you were twenty years old?
7. Do you snore? Does your partner say that your snoring keeps him or her awake?
8. Do you get out of breath when you climb two flights of stairs?
9. Do you avoid exercise because it is too hard to fit into your schedule?
10. Have you ever been mistaken for you spouse's parent, even though your ages are less than ten years apart?

If you answered yes to any of the above questions, you are in the pre-illness phase. You are not living a healthy and age-defying life. You are putting yourself at risk for disease, and the risk will increase as time goes by. This will not get better on its own. But you are the master of your own destiny and can change. You can change today. Do it for yourself by selecting only the foods that affirm health and go for an aerobic walk today. Don't worry about how many pounds you need to lose or how out of shape you are. Just take one day at a time. You can affect your health more than you realize!

Carbohydrates—The Fuel for the Fire

Fruits and vegetables are carbohydrates that are digested more slowly because of the presence of fiber. Plant cell walls are composed of fiber.

Fiber acts as a protective coating against digestive enzymes, slowing down the assimilation of carbohydrates. Snacks containing fiber are filling. Vegetables and fruits contain antioxidants, which help the body repair itself.

I often send my patients to dine at Primola, a cozy Italian restaurant on Second Avenue, slightly north of Bloomies. I love their homemade olive and tomato tapenade, which is served with celery instead of bread or breadsticks, so it makes a great savory appetizer without all the empty carbs that just fill you up. Their fish is suberbly prepared in the Mediterranean style and vegetables are generously presented family-style in a large bowl on the table.

Daily Aerobic Exercise

Exercise is essential to good health. It is critical that exercise become a habit if you are to reverse the pre-illness phase. The benefits of regular aerobic exercise extend far beyond just helping with weight loss and weight maintenance. Exercise causes our muscles to become stronger. The heart is a muscle and like every other muscle in the body it, too, becomes stronger with exercise. The coronary arteries, which supply blood to the heart, become more responsive and dilate to allow for improved circulation to the heart with regular exercise. The lungs become stronger when we breathe harder during exercise. The circulation to our skin is increased, supplying the cells with oxygen.

Even if you are out of shape and have not exercised in years, there is no reason why you cannot be physically fit. A recent study took middle-aged men, none of whom exercised on a regular basis, and put them on a regular aerobic exercise program. Within two months they returned to the level of fitness that they had had twenty years earlier. And they felt twenty years younger. This is amazing and should encourage anyone who has not been exercising to begin. Exercise is truly the fountain of youth! Celebrate the fact that you have the ability to move; there are people who do not have this gift and they would give anything to be able to exercise. You have this wonderful ability, therefore use it fully and encourage your body to become stronger and more agile.

The single most beneficial exercise for anyone, one that should be done throughout the day, and an exercise that I advise for all my patients, has to do with posture. I advise them as they are going about their daily routine to "keep your shoulders *back and down*." This simple movement aligns the spine, takes stress off the lower back, and opens the chest. Instantly you appear taller, slimmer, and more self-confident. You magically appear five pounds thinner! This is the posture associated with youth and vitality—make it your own.

NEW YORK CITY—A WALKERS' PARADISE

Central Park was the first landscaped public park in the United States. It is elegantly designed with magnificent old trees and other beautiful plants. Advocates of creating the park were primarily wealthy merchants and landowners, who long admired the public grounds of London and Paris, and wanted New York to have something comparable. In 1853, the City of New York acquired more than 700 acres of land in the center of Manhattan. At the time, the rough terrain between Fifth and Eighth avenues and 59th and 106th streets made it undesirable for private development.

In 1857, the Central Park Commission held the country's first landscape design contest and selected the "Greensward Plan" submitted by Frederick Law Olmsted, the park's superintendent at the time, and Calvert Vaux, an English-born architect. The designers sought to create a pastoral landscape in the English Romantic tradition. They added separate carriage drives, pedestrian walks, and equestrian paths, and designed more than forty bridges to eliminate grade crossings between the different routes. In 1863, the extension of the boundaries to 110th Street brought Central Park up to its current 843 acres. Originally created by the wealthy, Central Park is open and safe for everyone to enjoy. For bike riders, walkers, and runners, it offers a chance

(continued)

to be outside the city while being in the city. There are paths of varying lengths throughout the park. I suggest using these to progressively increase the length of your workout.

- Begin by briskly walking or slow-jogging around the Great Lawn Oval. This is a half mile in circumference. It is a wide and open expanse. This is a wonderful place to begin an aerobic program; when you are comfortable with one revolution, go around twice. When two revolutions are too easy, it's time to head up to change locales.
- When you have mastered the Great Lawn Oval, head for the Jacqueline Kennedy Onassis Reservoir Track. The flat track is 1.5 miles in circumference, circling a body of water that was once the water supply for Manhattan. The famous First Lady jogged this path daily. As you get stronger, work your way up to going around twice, for a 3-mile workout.
- The Lower Loop of the park is a circular path beginning at Fifty-ninth Street and going up to Seventy-second Street. It is 1.7 miles and offers both flat and gentle hills.
- The Big Loop circles all of Central Park and is 6.03 miles. Did you know that in the early days of the New York City Marathon, the runners went around the park four times, to equal 26 miles?

This is just a taste of what is available in New York City. But wherever you live, you can find open spaces for walking or jogging. In warmer climates, shopping malls are an ideal venue for brisk walking. They tend to be open early and are air-conditioned, and provide a good way to get out of the sun's harmful rays. By enlisting a partner to accompany you, you are giving this person a health gift! The two of you will have a great time. Or, if you need to use your walking time to reflect and meditate, enjoy this active alone time. Whatever your preference or location, just go out and walk. It will renew your body and spirit.

Scottsdale, Arizona, is a vacation destination for many New Yorkers. Scottsdale's terrain is dominated by the majestic Camelback Mountain, which does indeed look like a camel in repose. While visiting the home of friends in Scottsdale, I began my mornings with a hike along well-marked paths leading up to the top of the mountain. I was happy to note that a great number of retired people made a point of daily climbing Camelback in the cool mornings. And I will tell you that, although I consider myself to be a strong and active woman, those senior citizens passed me with ease going up the mountain! They were familiar with the paths and literally skipped past a city slicker like me! The beautiful Arizona landscape with the breathtaking red color of the rocks, purple shadows, a clear blue sky streaked with the sun's early rays, and a palette of wild flowers was not wasted on these fortunate individuals. I remain inspired by their joy in an early-morning climb!

Chapter Three

CALCIUM — THE MIRACLE MINERAL

Milk. Nature's most perfect food.

• • •

You may recall this advertising slogan from the Dairy Council. It turns out that they were right on the money, but they should have said, "*Calcium* is nature's most perfect food." It is not just milk but all dairy products that benefit us, providing the fat is removed. This is because all dairy products contain calcium. And calcium is very important for our health. In fact, it is essential.

Calcium and Bone Health

Everyone knows by now about the importance of adequate calcium intake to prevent bone loss, especially in women. Peak bone mass is achieved during the teenage years and, after that, the goal is to maintain what we have by weight-bearing activity and adequate calcium intake. Young men and women alike require 1,000 mg of calcium per day. After age fifty, the requirement rises to 1,200 mg per day. But the absorption of calcium is the tricky element, we can only absorb 500 mg at any one time, and the calcium needs vitamin D to be absorbed. This is important, because many calcium supplements have high amounts of calcium and can leave the false impression that a greater amount of calcium is being absorbed than is the case. Packaged foods also leave this impression; there are cereals that advertise that they supply 100 percent of the daily requirement of calcium. It doesn't help if they supply it but you can't absorb it!

Adding to the difficulty of absorption is the fact that certain nutrients also prevent the assimilation of calcium. These are iron and fiber. So, if you drink a glass of skim milk with a serving of steak or a high-fiber muffin, you will not absorb the 300 mg of calcium in the milk. You will absorb some calcium but you won't get the maximum present, because the nutrients compete for absorption.

Caffeine also prevents the absorption of calcium. That caffe skim latte in the morning doesn't give you all the calcium that you might think, so don't count this in your daily calcium tally. The key is to be aware of these interactions so that you are not deprived of your requirement. Remember, the requirement before age fifty years is 1,000 mg/day for men and women and, after age fifty, it rises to 1,200 mg/day.

DAILY CALCIUM REQUIREMENT

Children 4–8 years	800 mg calcium
Youth 9–18 years	1,300 mg calcium
Adults 19–50 years	1,000 mg calcium
Adults over 50 years	1,200 mg calcium
Pregnant or nursing women	1,200 mg calcium

Got Milk?

Fat-free is clearly preferred. Why waste calories on putting 2 percent milk in your coffee? Soy milk is not an ideal choice, either, because it is not a complete protein, as milk is, has extra calories, and does not give you as much calcium.

> *Keep milk cold at the back of the refrigerator, at 35°–40°F, not on a door shelf. Each 5°F rise in temperature shortens milk's shelf life because of bacterial growth.*

The sad fact is that teens are drinking half as much milk as they did thirty years ago. Milk has been replaced with newfangled drinks including designer bottled waters, exotic juices, iced teas, and soy beverages. But the saddest fact of all is the replacement of milk with carbonated sweetened beverages. When milk is replaced with carbonated beverages, the result is a loss from the diet of protein, calcium, magnesium, and vitamins A and D. There is an almost linear relationship between the rise in consumption of carbonated drinks and obesity in teens. Teenagers need to build bone mass that will last for a lifetime. Because of this, we have to look for new and creative ways to get the calcium we need every day. Space your intake of calcium during the day and also take a calcium supplement as an insurance policy.

Which Calcium Supplement Is Best?

Supplemental calcium comes in two forms: calcium carbonate and calcium citrate. Calcium carbonate must be taken with meals. This is also the type of calcium found in TUMS. By consuming this indigestion remedy, you are giving your bone density a boost. Calcium citrate may be taken any time—with or without food. I recommend that my patients take at bedtime a supplement of calcium citrate containing vitamin D.

Even if you receive your calcium requirement from food, I recommend adding a calcium supplement just to insure adequate intake. If you have trouble swallowing calcium tablets, as many people do, try another form of calcium. TUMS and calcium chews are popular, and easy for most people to consume. They contain calcium carbonate and must be taken with food for the calcium to be digested. Calcium citrate can be taken with or without food. Make sure that your calcium supplement also contains vitamin D, for optimal absorption.

You need to be aware of the amount of elemental calcium any supplement contains. The term "elemental calcium" refers to the amount of calcium in a supplement that is available for your body to absorb. Most calcium supplements list on the label the amount of elemental calcium. Some brands list only the total weight—in milligrams (mg)—of each tablet. This is the weight of the calcium, plus whatever may be bound to it—such as carbonate, citrate, lactate, or gluconate. For calcium, the % Daily Value (DV) is based on 1,000 mg of elemental calcium, so every 10 percent in the Daily Value column represents 100 mg of elemental calcium (0.10 × 1,000 mg = 100 mg). For example, if a calcium supplement has 60 percent Daily Value, it contains 600 mg of elemental calcium (0.60 × 1,000 mg = 600 mg). It is also important to note the serving size—the number of tablets you must take to get the % DV listed on the label.

When choosing a calcium supplement, check the label for the abbreviation USP. The best supplements meet the voluntary standards of the U.S. Pharmacopeia (USP) for quality, purity, and tablet disintegration or dissolution. Generic brands of calcium supplements are often cheaper than name brands. However, they may not meet voluntary standards for tablet disintegration. In other words, they may dissolve more slowly, which decreases their effectiveness. Avoid calcium supplements that contain bone meal or dolomite, as these may also contain toxic substances, such as lead, mercury, and arsenic. Check the label for "no added sugar." Chelated calcium tablets tend to be more expensive and really do not have any advantage over other types of calcium. Coral calcium is also marketed as superior calcium, which has not been proven.

Many of my patients love Viactiv Calcium Soft Chews—chewy little squares that taste like Kraft caramels and come in several dessertlike flavors. Although they are very sweet, two squares contain 100 percent of the Daily Value of calcium and include vitamins D and K. Each VI-ACTIV Calcium Soft Chew contains 500 mg of elemental calcium from 1,250 mg of calcium carbonate. (www.viactiv.com)

Calcium and Blood Pressure

Glimmerings of this important relationship began in 1982, when Dr. David A. McCarron noted that a diet low in dairy products increased a person's chance of developing high blood pressure.[1] A study of the entire population of the United States confirmed his hypothesis and revealed that the people who ate the least amount of dairy products had the highest blood pressures. In fact, the normal diet of the majority of United States doesn't meet the minimal requirement for adequate calcium. This led to a 1997 clinical trial, Dietary Approaches to Stop Hypertension, or the DASH trial, which showed that blood pressure could be lowered by a diet high in fruits, vegetables, and low-fat dairy products.[2] While fruits and vegetables lowered the blood pressure somewhat, it was the addition of dairy products that made the difference. The importance of maintaining an optimal blood pressure cannot be overstated. High blood pressure stresses the heart, strains the arteries, and increases the risk of heart attack and stroke. How remarkable that we can lower the risk for these terrible consequences simply by adding dairy products to our diets! I am constantly surprised that my patients who have high blood pressure have not been told anything about this relationship by their primary care physicians.

If you have high blood pressure, you should have a minimum of one dairy product at each meal. This can be easily accomplished by adding a glass of skim milk, 2 ounces of low-fat cheese, or a 6-ounce container of low-fat yogurt at each meal. This can be as vital as your taking your medication.

Marcia is a forty-seven-year-old divorced mother of two teenage sons who works as a museum curator. She was referred to me by her primary care doctor for weight reduction. When I first met Marcia, she was five foot three and weighed 160 pounds. Her cholesterol and blood pressure were elevated and she took medication for both of these conditions. On the positive side, she had a commitment to exercise and swam three times per week for the last twenty-five years. However, Marcia's diet was sadly deficient in the foods that she needed to control her blood pressure and cholesterol. Her typical breakfast was coffee and a croissant with butter, lunch was a sandwich, and dinner was often her sons' leftover pizza. These foods were the worst possible choices for someone with her health problems. In revamping Marcia's life, I suggested that she start a walk-run program, which she readily committed to. There is greater weight loss with walking or running than with swimming. For food, I suggested that she begin her day with a veg-

(continued)

etable omelet and a glass of skim milk. For a midmorning snack, she had some plain yogurt and fresh berries. (This reminded her of the summer she spent in France, where she began each morning with fresh raspberries and yogurt.) Lunch was a fruit salad with low-fat cottage cheese. I pointed out to Marcia that it was in her best interests to encourage her housekeeper to stop indulging her sons' pizza cravings, and to have her prepare a wholesome meal for them instead. Her housekeeper began preparing grilled fish or chicken with fresh herbs, two vegetables, and a salad for dinner. She set aside a portion of the meal for Marcia, who had a glass of skim milk with dinner and a calcium supplement prior to retiring.

The changes Marcia experienced were truly remarkable. She became a devoted runner, lost 40 pounds, and no longer required medication to control her blood pressure or cholesterol. Her health problems had been totally resolved by dietary changes. Even her sex life improved. She proudly showed me a bikini she had purchased for a vacation to France with her new boyfriend!

Calcium and Cancer Risk Reduction

Population studies indicate that a diet high in calcium lowers the risk for colon cancer. In both the Nurses Health Study, which included 88,000 women, and the Health Professionals Follow-up Study, with 47,300 men, people with the highest calcium intakes had the lowest rates of colon cancer.[3] There was an inverse risk of colon cancer, meaning that the more calcium consumed, the lower the risk for cancer. The way that calcium reduces colon cancer is by binding digestive acids that could potentially harm the cells of the colon lining. The cells of the colon are susceptible to damage by fatty acids and bile (produced by the body to digest dietary fat). If they are subjected to these acids on a regular basis (as is the case with a high-fat diet), the cells proliferate and polyps form. Colonic polyps are precancerous tissue. They are not cancers but, allowed to grow, may evolve into cancer. (This is why it is important for everyone to have a colonoscopy after fifty. As we age, the colon cells are more apt to form polyps. These are easily removed during a colonoscopy before they have a chance to become cancerous.) When digestive acids are bound to calcium, they are inactivated and rendered incapable of damaging the colon cells. Furthermore, when people prone to developing polyps consume high amounts of calcium, formation of polyps is reduced.[4]

If you have had colon cancer or colonic polyps, or have a family history of colon cancer, it is wise to lower the amount of fat in your diet and increase your calcium intake. The best way to do this is by incorporating low-fat dairy products and adding a calcium supplement.

Calcium and Weight Loss

Even more intriguing than the association of a reduction in blood pressure and cancer risk with calcium is the association of calcium with weight loss. The relation between calcium and body weight was first noted more than twenty years ago in the National Health and Nutrition Examination Survey. This study of the nutritional habits of the entire United States reported that the slimmest people had the highest intakes of calcium. Since there was no known mechanism for how calcium kept people thin, the finding was written off as pure chance. When the study was repeated ten years later, it was found that not only did the slimmest people have the highest calcium intakes, but the heaviest people had the lowest calcium intakes! Now, this got researchers' attention: Perhaps there *could* be a connection between calcium and weight.

A study at the University of Tennessee found that when fat cells were exposed to a calcium-rich environment, they broke down fat much more rapidly than when they were in a calcium-depleted environment.[5] That was a very interesting finding but it was done in a Petri dish, not in human clinical trials. The reasons for the cells behaving in this manner are believed to date back to our prehistoric origins.[6] In ancient times, our diets had much more calcium, due to the consumption of nuts, tubers, and roots grown in calcium-rich soil. Examination of the skeletons of prehistoric man shows bones with high amounts of calcium. Some researchers estimate the ancient diet had two to three times the calcium consumed today. In light of this, it may be that the body may respond to a low calcium intake as a state of starvation, causing it to hold on to fat stores more closely. Of course, this is all speculative.

What about real people and calcium? Can calcium really help them lose weight? In 2004, a published study showed that this was indeed the case.[7] This weight-loss study, also from the University of Tennessee, divided overweight subjects into three groups. Each group was restricted by the same amount of calories, and the proportions of fat, carbohydrate, and protein were the same for each group. But they differed in the amount of calcium in their diets: One group had 1,200 to 1,300 mg of dairy (food-derived) calcium per day, another had 800 mg of supplemental calcium per day, and the third received no additional calcium. What do you suppose happened? The group that received 1,200 mg of dairy calcium *lost 70 percent more weight* than did the calcium-depleted group! And the group that consumed dairy products lost more weight than the group that got the same amount of calcium from supplements.

This tells us two very important things:

1. Calcium can help us lose weight.
2. There may be an as yet undiscovered factor in dairy foods that works with calcium to aid in fat breakdown.

It is a well-known fact that women frequently go on diets. When they do, they often eliminate dairy foods in an effort to save calories. This is not only bad for their bone health, but counterproductive from a weight-loss perspective.

Cut your calories but don't cut your calcium!

Dairy products are also terrific sources of protein. The amino acids in milk are especially helpful to our bodies. Milk contains *branched chain amino acids.* Branched chain amino acids build muscles. The benefit of dairy products to a weight-loss program is both enhanced weight loss along with increased lean muscle mass. This does not mean that you will build weight lifter–type muscles but that you will look sleeker and fit.

Including 1,200 mg per day of dairy calcium in your diet plan has been proven to reduce the size of your waistline. In the University of Tennessee study, this is exactly what happened: In the study, the people on the low-calcium diet lost 5 percent of their belly fat, while people on high-calcium diets lost 14 percent of their belly fat. Milk products caused *three times* more fat to be lost from the waist! As discussed earlier, an increasing waistline is the hallmark of middle age.

A frequent concern that my patients voice before beginning a diet is that they fear losing weight from their faces. They do not want to look "gaunt." On my high-calcium plan, this will not occur because it is precisely middle-aged belly fat that is eliminated first. You will see your waistline become svelte, and fit into clothes that have been lingering in the back of your closet!

Start the plan right now by having a low-fat, calcium-rich snack. Don't fall into the trap of waiting until Monday, or after the holidays, or a week from next Tuesday. The best time to start a healthy eating plan is NOW!

What if I Am Lactose Intolerant?

A segment of the population does have difficulty digesting milk. Some are lactose intolerant, and some cannot tolerate casein, milk protein. Heredity plays a role: Many people who can't tolerate milk and milk products come from Asian, African, Mediterranean, or Jewish backgrounds. Dairy foods have gotten a bad reputation in recent years, but the truth is that the vast majority of people can tolerate some dairy.

Lactose intolerance occurs when the body lacks the enzyme *lactase,* necessary for the metabolism of the sugar, *lactose,* found in milk. Usually this is not a problem because you may simply take a pill with the enzyme prior to consuming the dairy product. Also most people who are lactose intolerant are able to tolerate some kinds of dairy: The enzyme cultures that create yogurt and most hard cheeses also break down lactose, so that these foods are usually safe. Soy products are an excellent source of both calcium and protein, and are low in fat. Soy cheeses are absolutely delicious and often have as much calcium as dairy cheeses. Canned salmon and sardines are high in calcium because of the bones present, though of course you must eat the bones to obtain this benefit. Vegetables such as kale and collards contain lesser amounts of calcium, often dependent upon the soil in which they are grown. I do not recommend calcium-enriched juices, as they tend to be too high in calories and sugar.

Yogurt

Yogurt is a wonderful and versatile calcium source. It may be made from cow's milk or goat's milk. Some people who are allergic to the proteins in cow's milk may tolerate goat's milk better. I suggest that you choose one that is low fat or preferably fat free, to keep your intake of saturated fat at a minimum. Both types of yogurt contain high amounts of calcium, vitamin A, and protein. Do not choose a highly processed yogurt with "fruit on the bottom." There really isn't any fruit on the bottom but, rather, highly sweetened preserves! Instead, choose a preservative-free plain yogurt and add your own fresh fruit. Yogurt should be made from Grade A skim milk and live active yogurt cultures. Many of the current products called yogurt do not have live active yogurt cultures; the cultures may have been alive originally, but overprocessing kills them. Look for a high amount of protein and calcium in your yogurt.

I recommend Fage Total 0%, the number-one-selling yogurt in Greece. This delicious yogurt comes in three varieties: 0% fat, 2% fat, and full fat. Of course, I prefer my patients to use the fat-free variety, which is made from skimmed cow's milk and live yogurt culture. One 6.5-ounce serving contains 80 calories, 15 g of protein, 6 g of carbohydrate, and 150 mg of calcium. It is great for breakfast, lunch, or as a nutritious, healthy snack. (www.fageusa.com)

Another good yogurt product is made by Stonyfield Farms. They make an organic plain low-fat variety that is 99 percent fat free, but avoid the fruit flavors, which are loaded with sugar. (www.stonyfield.com)

Look at the ingredient list: If it sounds like it was made in a Laboratory instead of a dairy, or if you can't pronounce it, don't buy it!

How Can I Find Healthy Low-Fat Cheeses?

Cheese should be hormone free, antibiotic free, and come from grass-fed animals. The best choice is organic cheese from grass-fed cows. These cheeses will contain omega-3 fat and conjugated linoleic acid (CLA), which is absent in cows that are fed in feed pens. As I have explained, the omega-3 fats are anti-inflammatory and CLA may protect against cancer.

There is a difference in the composition of the milk depending on its animal source:

- Goats
- Sheep or Ewes
- Cows
- Buffalo

In some cultures, cheese is even made from the milk of reindeer, mares, camels, and yaks. The best choice is organic cheese made with cow's or sheep's milk, according to your taste.

What Is Low Fat?

The FDA defines "low fat" as being a food that contains 3 grams or less of fat per serving. It is optimal to aim for minimizing *saturated* fat. The definition of low saturated fat is 1 gram or less per serving. Saturated fat is found mainly in animal products. So one 8-ounce container of low-fat yogurt, for example, contains 3 grams of fat, of which 2 grams are saturated fat. Thus, low-fat yogurt, while low in total fat, is not low in saturated fat, per FDA definition.

An excellent cheese choice is Jarlsberg Lite, from Norway, made from cow's milk: A 1-ounce serving has 70 calories, 3.5 g of total fat, 2.0 g of saturated fat, 9 g of protein, and 20 percent calcium. Have it on a slice of apple for a nutritious snack.

Did you know that Coach, which makes trendy handbags and leather accessories, also makes a great low-fat goat cheese? In 1983, the Cahn family bought an abandoned dairy farm outside New York City. Two years into the project, they sold Coach Leatherware to Sara Lee Corp, moved to the farm full time, and now make Coach Farm fresh and aged goat cheeses. Try the Low-Fat Black Pepper Stick, a delicious cheese made with goat's milk from which Coach Farm removes more than half the fat, and which is rolled in black pepper. A 1-ounce serving has only 45 calories, 3 g of total fat, 1.5 g of saturated fat, and 4 grams of protein. (www.coachfarm.com)

VEGETABLES WITH CALCIUM

When considering obtaining calcium from vegetable sources, keep in mind the bioavailability of the calcium. Calcium bioavailability is decreased by the amount of fiber and iron in the food. Iron competes with calcium for absorption, and fiber can block digestion of the calcium. Dairy products remain your best calcium source!

FOOD	AMOUNT OF CALCIUM	BIOAVAILABILITY
Broccoli, ½ cup	35 mg	good
Cabbage, ½ cup	79 mg	good
Kale, ½ cup	47 mg	good
Edamame (soybeans), ¼ cup	65 mg	good
Spinach, ½ cup	122 mg	fair
Beans, dried, ½ cup	50 mg	poor

Although green leafy vegetables are good sources of calcium, you would need to eat 5 cups of broccoli to equal the calcium in 1 cup of milk. Similarly, you would need to consume 3 tablespoons of sesame seeds, 8 medium-size sardines, 4.5 ounces of canned salmon, 1½ cups of cooked kale, or ¾ cup of roasted almonds for that amount of calcium.

The Chinese food guide, The Pagoda, offers these dairy equivalents, because Asian diets tend to be low in dairy products, which may account for their high incidence of osteoporosis.

Note that these will not have the same protein, essential amino acids, or CLA as dairy-derived calcium, and that the mineral is not as easily absorbed:

- Almonds
- Bok choy
- Broccoli
- Kale
- Salmon
- Sardines
- Sesame seeds

What About Soy?

Soybeans contain more protein than any other legume. Depending on the form, soy products can also be a great source of calcium. The calcium in soy milk, however, is not as readily available for the body to use as it is in cow's milk.

- *Edamame* are soybeans in the pod or shelled, popular in sushi restaurants. They are popular in chic New York restaurants as an alternative to the ubiquitous bread basket. Rich in vitamins A and B, and high in calcium, they make a great snack. They are available in the whole pod (which I prefer) or shelled in the frozen food section of the supermarket. They are calcium rich and make a wonderful snack when steamed or boiled. They are also good finger food.
- *Soy milk* is made by cooking and crushing soybeans, then straining the liquid. There are flavorings added to this, usually including sweeteners.
- *Soy nuts* are toasted soybeans. They are delicious in salads or sprinkled over broccoli or any other vegetables.

- *Tofu* is made from soy milk. It is high in protein: 4 ounces have 12 g of protein, similar to cheese. Whether or not it will have calcium depends on the method of preparation. Tofu is made by adding calcium or magnesium salt to soy milk, forming a curd. If the calcium salt is added, the tofu becomes a good calcium source. Check the label!

Note: Many vegetarian and vegan restaurants will add tofu to their dishes if requested, especially stir-fries and salads. Candle 79, on Seventy-ninth Street off Lexington Avenue, is one that I frequently recommend. In fact, I have their vegan cookbook in my office, called *The Candle Café Cookbook*, which is filled with many innovative tofu recipes. To stick with my diet plan just avoid the recipes that call for grains and starches.

The best sources of calcium are milk, yogurt, and cheese. About 72 percent of the calcium in the U.S. food supply comes from dairy foods.

CALCULATING YOUR CALCIUM

PRODUCT	CALCIUM MG/SERV	# SERVINGS PER DAY	TOTAL MG/DAY
Yogurt, 0% fat	150	2	300
Skim milk	300	2	600
Low-fat cheese	150	2	300

The above will give you a ballpark figure for estimating calcium contents totaling 1,200 mg, so you can make sure that your daily intake of this fabulous mineral is optimal.

(continued)

CALCIUM SCORECARD

Keep a running tally throughout the day. Make it into a game. Your goal is to get to 12 points.

For example, yogurt is 4 points. Milk is 3 points. Each serving of low-fat cheese is 1.5 points.

When you get to 12 points, you win! You win stronger bones and a thinner body.

SINGLE SERVING	CALCIUM/MG	% DAILY VALUE*
MILK		
Milk (skim), 8 ounces	302	30%
CHEESE		
Low-fat cottage cheese, 1 cup	15	2%
Feta cheese, 1 ounce	140	14%
Grated Parmesan cheese, 1 tablespoon	69	7%
Swiss cheese, 1 ounce	27	3%
YOGURT		
Low-fat yogurt, 8 ounces	415	42%
VEGETABLES		
Broccoli (cooked), 1 cup	178	18%
Spinach (cooked), ½ cup	120	12%

Source: American Osteoporosis Foundation

*Percentage is based on the daily value of 1,000 mg of calcium. Calcium requirements will vary for those 9–18 and men and women ages 51-plus.

WATER AS A SOURCE OF CALCIUM

Did you know that you can get extra calcium just by drinking water?

Hydration is important to anyone attempting to lose weight and it can also give an extra calcium boost, if you choose mineral water. Perrier has approximately 60 mg of calcium per liter and San Pellegrino has approximately 120 mg of calcium per liter while Sanfaustino has approximately 400 mg of calcium per liter! I advise my patients to forgo the alcohol and make these their cocktails of choice. They are not called mineral water for nothing!

There are so many benefits from calcium that it really is a miracle mineral. Calcium lowers blood pressure and the risk for cardiovascular disease, lowers the risk for colon cancer (the second leading cause of cancer death in the United States), maintains our skeletal mass, and keeps us slim. It is readily available, inexpensive, and present in a wide variety of delicious foods. If you want to lose weight and keep it off, add more low-fat dairy products to your diet. Weight loss will be easier, you will lose weight from unhealthy abdominal stores, and your total health will improve.

_____

Chapter Four

DR. KLAUER'S DIET PLAN

*Whatever you can do, or dream you can,
begin it. Boldness has genius, power and
magic in it.*

—GOETHE

•   •   •

You know it's time. You know you need to do it. You know you want it.
When you look in the mirror, you don't like what you see and you don't
like the way your clothes fit. The hardest part is just getting started. You
have already taken the first positive step by purchasing this book. Now you
need to arrange your life so that your weight-loss success is guaranteed.

Getting Started

1. *Set a start date.* Put it in writing to make it official—circle the
   date on your calendar or designate it in your PDA. If you have
   planned your husband's surprise birthday dinner for fifty
   friends for tomorrow night, it is probably best to wait until the
   next day before you begin. But be aware of the tendency that all
   of us have, to procrastinate. The sooner you get started, the
   sooner you will reach your goal weight. Think of this as your
   most important appointment; you must not miss or postpone it.
   This date is an appointment for your health and for your life.

2. *Get organized.* Go through your cupboard and refrigerator and throw away (do not eat!) any foods that could be triggers for you to fall off the plan. Get rid of crackers, cookies, and any processed foods. Throw out all those herbs that have been collecting dust. It is surprising to me, the number of dried herbs in pantries. Fresh herbs have high antioxidant properties and numerous health benefits. In many countries, herbs are considered medicines. But when herbs are kept for too long, they become stale and lose their potency. Make it a rule to use only the freshest herbs. You will be astonished at the increase in cupboard space. Throw out oils you haven't purchased recently. They are now rancid.

3. *Go shopping.* Replace bad foods with good ones. The foods in your home should be foods that will help you satisfy cravings without adding pounds to your frame: fresh vegetables; high-calcium foods, such as low-fat yogurt and low-fat cheese; and omega-3 eggs. Purchase a case of mineral water, and fresh limes or lemons, to ensure hydration. Buy fresh herbs; they add flavor and complexity to food. Buy a small bottle of extra-virgin olive oil and transfer it to a dark, tightly lidded container. You want everything that you eat to benefit your health, so freshness is essential.

Danger Foods to Get Rid Of

- Anything that contains partially hydrogenated corn oil or fructose corn syrup
- Crackers, cookies, cake mixes, dried pasta, dried fruits (raisins, apricots, apples, etc.), powdered drink mixes (orange juice substitute, iced tea or lemonade mix), "instant" anything
- Dried herbs
- Vegetable oil blends, and even possibly your olive oil, if not fresh. Olive oil oxidizes over time; it has gone stale in most homes that I have visited.
- Ice cream, sherbet, sorbet, frozen yogurt, Popsicles, and any other frozen desserts, even if they are low calorie. Frozen waffles, muffins, or ready-to-heat hors d'oeuvres need to go. Don't save any frozen dinners "for an emergency"—even if they are low-carb and advertised as being part of a diet plan.

- Candy, even if it is very elegantly packaged and was given to you as a gift. Re-gift it—pass it on to someone else. Avoid diet candy also, which is usually loaded with preservatives and sorbitol, a sugar alcohol that reinforces your cravings.
- Diet carbonated beverages
- Any food that contains ingredients that are unpronounceable. Only the freshest and best foods should be included in your life.

Jane, who has a high-profile New York social life, decided that she wanted to become healthier and slimmer in anticipation of her sixtieth birthday, which was six months in the future. She readily incorporated lifestyle changes that I suggested: She changed her eating habits easily and began walking in Central Park daily with her husband. It was wonderful to watch as Jane's health improved and her body became stronger and fit. Excess pounds were shed, her cholesterol became normal, and Jane looked and felt wonderful. But because of the nature of her husband's professional position, companies were constantly sending expensive gifts to their home. Often they received huge cookie tins from Fauchon, Godiva chocolates, La Maison du Chocolat truffles, and other sinful sweets, especially at Christmastime. Jane decided that she had to get these out of the house to resist the temptation for her, and for her husband and children. So, whenever the elegant but weight-promoting treats arrived, Jane immediately gave them to her doorman, who really appreciated them. Over the next few months, Jane noticed that her doorman was getting progressively chubbier. As she was losing weight, he was putting on pounds from all these sugary, high-carb desserts.

When you open your SubZero side-by-side, as my patients often do, the first thing you should see is a beautiful glass bowl filled with crisp and delicious cut-up veggies immersed in ice water so they don't oxidize. Replace the mixture every two days so it stays fresh. Include carrots, cucumbers, broccoli, cauliflower, crunchy things like red, yellow, and green peppers, and jicama. Vegetables are low in calories and loaded with antioxidants that can help build and repair your tissues. This should be your new daily snack.

Don't forget to give yourself a reward occasionally. Do something for yourself that celebrates who you are. By this I mean, if you enjoy collecting art, buy yourself a painting; if you love music, sign up for a concert series; and so on. Stop rewarding yourself with food.

A top literary figure in New York City keeps her beautiful figure by buying tickets to a fantastic Broadway play for the evening of the date that she starts her diet. She follows her diet all day knowing that she will see a wonderful show that night as her reward.

A young attorney, who lost over 100 pounds, gave herself the reward of new pair of Jimmy Choos for each 10 pounds lost. This young woman, an avid fashionista, realized that it made little sense to purchase an entire expensive wardrobe until she had reached her goal, but shoes were her "retail therapy." She satisfied her cravings for gorgeous clothes, as well as for food, by hitting the shoe department.

Of course, $700 shoes can be an expensive treat. Consider continuing a more reasonable and cost-effective reward policy throughout your diet with a week's-end bonus of a therapeutic massage, a new lipstick, a great book—anything but food!

In my experience, the people who succeed in losing weight (and in life) have a goal, a plan for getting where they want to be, and stay focused. These characteristics describe the majority of my patients, and these are the characteristics that have enabled them to attain their opulent lifestyle.

Consider the inspiring story of Margot, a top financial analyst in New York. She began her career as an assistant to a man who spent a great deal of time on the golf course. Since this was her first job out of college, she made a point of trying to learn as much as she could about the industries that her boss covered so that she could field the questions that her boss's clients had while he enjoyed his golf game. Quietly, she set about to gain as much knowledge as she could, often staying late at work and reading reports. In time, she realized that she knew the industry as well as, if not better than, the man she was covering for. As you might guess, her keen observations enabled her to be hired away and now she has surpassed her mentor in terms of income and reputation. When Margot decided that her weight was not what she wanted it to be, she applied the same strategy: She consulted me, learned what she needed to know about nutrition and exercise, hired a trainer, and followed her diet plan to a T. She didn't deviate, procrastinate, complain, or waiver—she had a goal, and she planned and focused.

People with this mind-set get results because they are able to stay focused on the endpoint. Then it all comes down to a matter of time, however long it takes, for they reach their goal. Sure, there are times when it is tough, but have a goal and a good plan, and you will succeed. See yourself as that superachiever!

My plan has everything that your body needs to stay healthy and to lose weight at an optimal rate. You are eliminating food with unnecessary calories and harmful fat. Most of my patients say that once they are on the plan they are not hungry and feel more energetic than they have felt in years. You, too, will feel the same way.

The preliminary phase of this plan is the most challenging, not so much because of the foods involved but because you will be required to change your current bad eating habits. Human beings are programmed to resist change. Even when something may be harmful to us, we resist changing it. But there comes a time when all the old excuses must be left behind. We must accept the challenge of changing our behavior, whether portion size or type of food, or both, is the problem. Changing your behavior is like moving into a new house; at first it feels unfamiliar and it takes some time to get the settings in the shower just right. But it's a good move if our old house is falling apart and its plumbing is in desperate need of an overhaul. So change we must, because the benefits of moving into a new and magnificent place of health far outweigh the discomfort involved in changing unhealthy old habits.

One of my patients, Belinda, exemplified this transformation. Once she started following my plan, and began to feel better and lose the extra weight she was carrying around, she recognized how destructive her old lifestyle had been. She was very grateful to me for showing her how to enjoy tasting good food again, instead of shoveling down anything that was served to her. She started eating healthy food without feeling deprived. In Belinda's own words, "I don't know how I fell into having this lifeless and pointless food." Lifeless and pointless, indeed.

If You Must Eat Out . . .

Even once your pantry and refrigerator are in gear for your beginning the Klauer Plan, you need to be prepared for the fact that you will not always eat at home. This is how my patients cope with restaurant dining:

Power Breakfasts

Many of my patients have breakfast meetings in restaurants. The most popular "power breakfast" spot in New York is the Regency Hotel; many high-profile deals have been consummated during breakfast here. Most restaurants will not have omega-3 eggs since they are more expensive than regular eggs. This is the case with the Regency Hotel; however, at least they do have organic eggs. An ideal choice is an egg-white omelet with low-fat cheese and vegetables. You must specify that it not be made with butter, and only a small amount of olive oil. The usual serving size for berries in restaurants is 1 cup, more than is recommended during the initial phase. Just eat half of the berries.

The Manhattan Lunch Scene

The trick to "lunching" is to have a good breakfast and then a light snack prior to lunch. Morning meetings can push the lunch hour to a later time, leading to overeating to assuage low blood glucose. I advise sparkling mineral water as your beverage of choice.

Follow these lunch rules and you will not have a problem:

1. Do not arrive at a luncheon hungry. Have a light snack, such as a piece of low-fat cheese or some turkey, just prior to lunch.
2. Drink only mineral water with lemon or lime.
3. Never touch the bread basket or dessert.
4. Always leave something on your plate. The Clean Plate Club is to be avoided at all costs.

If your lunch date is business, the point is to stay focused on the business project and not on the food. If the lunch purpose is social, the same principle applies—focus on being with your friend and not just food. The setting may be beautiful, the service and presentation superb, and the food itself may be delicious, but it is still never just about the food.

In Manhattan, where you go for lunch and where you sit are subtle clues as to social standing. At the Four Seasons Grill Room, for many, it is a tradition to be seen rather than to sup on the fine food; 21 is another popular eatery where business men and women go, and expect a specific table in the Bar Room. These legendary dining rooms are filled to capacity at lunchtime with New York's most accomplished movers and shakers. Each of these power scenes will accommodate the lunch rules that I have set forth. They will bring bottled mineral water to your table, provide a crudités plate, grill fish or chicken by lightly brushing with olive oil, eliminate any butter, substitute a vegetable for a potato listed on the menu, and, in effect, do things your way. That is the goal.

At dinner, follow the same plan as for lunch, and you can't go wrong.

You can go anywhere, even Manhattan's most intimidating restaurants, with the plan I've provided you with. All you have to do is make up your mind in advance and ask for what you want. I recommend that you add a site like www.menupages.com to your computer "favorites"—you can then check out the restaurant menu online and decide what you will buy in advance.

Are you ready to slim down?

The Jump-Start

This three-day program gets your metabolism into high gear. You will lose weight very quickly and dramatically. The magnitude of your excess weight will determine how much weight you will lose. For example, someone who is 50 pounds overweight will lose more than someone with 15 pounds to lose.

Men lose weight faster than women due to their greater muscle mass. If you are starting the diet with your husband, wife, or partner, do not compare your weights. You will just get discouraged. As a matter of fact, don't compare your weight with that of your dieting best friend either, as she or he has an entirely different metabolism. This plan is about you and gaining control of your health and weight. Focus on your own goal.

If your mind-set is such that an immediate result is what will motivate you, the jump-start portion of the plan is ideal for you. Your silhouette will be slimmer, your belly flatter, and you will feel better about how you look. Just eat only the items that are recommended. Do not deviate and do not add anything to this menu plan. It is only for three days!

LOSING THE BLOAT

Every cell in your body needs sodium to work properly. It is essential for the healthy function of nerve and muscle—including your heart muscle. The problem with sodium is that most of us consume far more than we need and it causes water retention. Salt is present in just about all packaged foods and all restaurant food. I suggest that you eliminate cooking with salt and, if you need a pinch for flavor, you can add it at the table. Once you have gotten rid of it for a while, you won't miss it. And you definitely won't miss the water retention that salt causes!

The symptoms of bloating are visible swelling, especially of the stomach, breasts, face, hands, ankles, and feet. When you consume excessive salt at a meal, it takes about three days to get rid of the excessive water weight in the body. It can also make you dizzy, which can be a problem in older people. As we age, the small subunits of the kidney, called nephrons, decline in number. Therefore, sodium is not as easily eliminated as we age.

Daily Sodium Guideline: 2,300 mg per day (USDA); 1,500 mg per day (Institute of Medicine)

Prepared, prepackaged, frozen, and other processed foods tend to contain high levels of sodium. Avoiding these and tasting your food before reaching for the salt shaker make a big difference in retention of fluid. For the three-day jump-start program, avoid salt entirely.

FLAVORFUL SUBSTITUTES FOR SALT

Try to use fresh herbs at all times.

Thyme	Bay leaves	Caraway
Dill weed	Saffron	Tarragon
Peppermint	Paprika	Rosemary
Basil	Parsley	Fresh garlic
Onion	Lemon or lime juice	Salt-free herb and spice mixes

A number of factors, including heat, humidity, and exercise, can place extra demands on your body's fluid needs. When the temperature rises, you may need to pay special attention to your fluid intake to replace what you sweat out, and to prevent heat cramps, heat exhaustion, or heatstroke:

- Drink 20 ounces of water (about 2½ cups) two or three hours before exercising.
- Consume another 10 ounces of water about 15 minutes before starting.
- During your workout, swig 10 ounces about every 15 minutes.
- After exercising, drink 20 ounces for every pound you lose working out.

Fluid retention can be eliminated with an appropriate diet. Exercise will help flush surplus fluid out of the body. If you are retaining fluids, as soon as you have finished exercising, you will need to urinate.

Refined carbohydrates contribute to fluid retention, along with certain food allergies. The most common cause of excess fluid retention is usually salt intake. Many of your salt habits have to do with the way you grew up, and your cultural background. Some cuisines are loaded with salty condiments and seasonings. For example, Chinese, Indian, Thai, Mexican, and Arabic cooking tend to be high in sodium and spices.

Your Jump-Start Schedule

The jump-start is a radical high-protein diet and should only be followed at the very beginning of this plan for three days, maximum. It will get off the extra bloat, allow you to break down fat quickly, and preserve your lean muscle mass. You must drink 2 to 3 quarts of water throughout each day, which will help reduce puffiness and inflammation.

Begin your exercise regimen of one hour per day. If the hour is impossible for you to do, do half an hour. If you cannot do half an hour all at once, split it into segments. But you must begin to move! The body that holds your spirit was not designed to be inactive. Walk as much as possible, using physical activity to suppress hunger.

BREAKFAST:
One omega-3 egg prepared without butter or oil. The egg may be boiled
or scrambled with a small amount of olive oil brushed onto the pan.
(80 calories)
8 ounces plain low-fat yogurt   (80 calories)
1 cup of green tea
1 large glass of water

MORNING SNACK:
2 ounces of low-fat cheese, such as Jarlsberg Lite, Finlandia Lite Swiss
(150 calories)
Several glasses of water spaced over the course of the morning

LUNCH:
1 (4-ounce) can of tuna or salmon, drained, with lemon and pepper. One
of the best is Tonno tuna, which is packed in olive oil and is a solid
light tuna, not white. (White tuna is higher in mercury than the
light.) It has 196 calories per 3-ounce can; draining it reduces the
calorie count to 150.   (150 calories)
A large glass of water

AFTERNOON SNACK:
8 ounces of low-fat calcium-enriched cottage cheese with ½ cup of raw
cauliflower or broccoli spears   (200 calories)
Several glasses of water over the course of the afternoon

DINNER:

2 cups of salad greens with 1 tablespoon of Ginger Soy Dressing (see
   page 188)

4 ounces of broiled or grilled fish or shellfish (may be brushed lightly
   with olive oil). Shellfish could be shrimp, king crabmeat, sea or bay
   scallops, and even lobster.

A ½ cup serving of broccoli, spinach, green beans, or asparagus. Vegetables should be steamed and topped with lemon juice only.

                                                    (485 calories total)

A large glass of water

BEFORE RETIRING:

8 ounces of plain low-fat yogurt   (80 calories)

Total calories: 1,225
Total protein: 105 grams
Total calcium: 1,300 mg

The three days that you invest in this will have a big payoff when you
step on the scale. I also suggest this plan for my Park Avenue socialite
patients who need to fit into a body-revealing dress within a few days.
The reason why this radical approach works is carbohydrates cause water retention—eliminate these, exercise, drink lots of water, and you will
see an immediate effect.

> *You should not kid yourself into thinking that you have lost a lot
> of excess fat; you have lost some fat but what mainly has been
> lost is water weight. To lose significant fat you must follow a bal-
> anced eating plan for a longer period of time.*

Once you have finished your three-day jump-start, it's time to enter
phase 1 of the plan proper.

Phase 1—The Get-It-Done Phase

The plan is composed of two phases. Phase 1 is more restrictive and provides for efficient weight loss. My patients are "results oriented," they want to see a change and they want it yesterday! Their "Get it done!" attitude serves them well in this phase. They don't waste time; they do what needs to be done. Phase 1 gets those unsightly pounds off quickly but without any nutritional deprivation. During phase 1, your body receives optimal nutrition; in fact, most people get the best nutrition in their lives from phase 1. There are no processed foods, no foods high in saturated fat, no empty-calorie sodas, and no alcohol.

You should feel free to continue with phase 1 for as long as necessary to get your weight within 5 pounds of your goal weight if you are a woman or 7 pounds if you are a man; there is nothing about this phase that can harm your body.

> If you have not seen a doctor in a while, are more than 30 pounds overweight, or have medical issues—consult your doctor before beginning this diet. This is just common sense.

I suggest moving to phase 2 as you near your goal because this allows you to gradually introduce new foods to your diet and thereby prevent weight regain. After losing a significant amount of weight, it takes the metabolism a period of time to "get used to" the new body weight. I tell my patients that they don't really own the new weight for approximately six to nine months. This is because the body has not adjusted to the new, lower weight and, if extra calories are added too quickly to the diet plan, they are quickly stored as fat. If you add new foods slowly, you allow the body time to adapt.

I have included a sample menu for the first week. If you want to have the foods for day 1 on day 3, that is fine. You can also exchange lunches for dinners and vice versa. Although you are free to switch around the meal plans, I advise against eating the same lunch or dinner repeatedly. Give yourself variety to avoid becoming bored. This will make it easier to stick with your plan.

The Main Principles

1. *Get your 1,200 mg of calcium daily.* Studies have shown a greater weight-loss benefit with dairy calcium than with calcium supplements. Dairy products provide the complete protein, B vitamins, and minerals that the body needs.

2. *Upgrade your protein sources.* Your sources for protein during the first phase are fish, poultry, eggs, and dairy *only*. This is because these are high-quality proteins. The type of fat associated with protein is crucial to its effect within the body. Meat is linked with saturated fat, and high amounts of saturated fat are harmful to the body. In contrast, fish is linked to omega-3 fat, a cardio-protective and anti-inflammatory fat that has great benefit to the body. Omega-3 fat has been shown to improve mood and may even prevent the mental decline associated with aging. I realize that not all people like fish, so they can substitute lean turkey or chicken with the skin removed. A new source for omega-3 fat is eggs. Formerly, eggs were to be avoided by anyone with elevated cholesterol. Due to an innovative idea to feed chickens flaxseed, which is high in omega-3 fat, the egg yolks from flax-fed chickens have become a concentrated source of omega-3 fat. Choose only low-fat or nonfat dairy foods.

3. *Practice prevention eating.* In order to stick to the plan, you must eat all the meals and every snack. Even if you are not feeling hungry, eat the snacks anyway. This is what I call prophylactic, or prevention, eating. You eat before you are hungry, so that you never become overly hungry. Allowing yourself to become ravenous is a recipe for disaster—it will become easy to give in to temptation. When you eat frequent small meals, your blood glucose remains in a steady range and you feel more energetic throughout the day.

WHAT ABOUT EGGS AND CHOLESTEROL?

While in the past we were urged to consume no more than 3 to 4 eggs per week because of the cholesterol present within the yolk of the egg (213 mg), now it appears that eggs do not have as much impact on the blood cholesterol as was feared. The American Heart Association no longer makes a recommendation about how many egg yolks can be eaten per week. They do, however, recommend a limit of two egg yolks per week for people at high risk or who have heart disease.

Omega-3 eggs are sold in most supermarkets and are labeled prominently, "omega-3 eggs." Omega-3 eggs are readily available throughout the U.S., but have various name brands. The brands found in the New York region are: Country Hen, Eggland's Best, and Nellie's. These eggs cost more but nonetheless are inexpensive sources of high quality protein and good fat. Each egg will contain approximately 150 mg of omega-3 fat.

As an alternative, you can just have egg whites and skip the yolk. Egg white is pure protein. Avoid egg substitutes, as these are not as good as the real thing and many varieties contain preservatives and added sodium.

Day 1

Begin your day with a large glass of water and with an aerobic workout of one hour. Aerobic exercise is exercise that causes your heart to beat faster and your breathing to become more rapid. You should sweat; this is normal. If you cannot carry on a conversation, you are working too hard. If this is the case, just slow down but don't stop exercising. The type of exercise that you choose is up to you.

Begin with walking because of its many proven benefits:

- It is easy to do.
- Almost anyone can do it.
- No special equipment is needed.
- It is a weight-bearing activity, so it makes your bones stronger.

Whoever Has the Most Toys Wins
Get yourself a pedometer. My patients love gadgets, gizmos, and electronics. So I often send them on a mission to Niketown on East Fifty-seventh Street to go shopping for a pedometer. This little device will tell you exactly how many steps you have taken toward your goal and will help you keep pushing to your eventual target number of steps a day. You will be walking more, which is the main objective. A good pedometer costs around ten dollars. It could be the best ten dollars you ever spent. Of course, some of my male patients end up buying the Triax Elite for three hundred dollars, which gives you a digital transmission of your heart rate and pace information for your every step, but the ten-dollar models work just fine. Pedometers are worn on the hip and, based on your body's movements, will count your steps. When you enter your stride length, the pedometer will calculate your distance walked and with your weight it can calculate the approximate number of calories burned. If you increase your number of steps consistently, you will have greater improvement in weight, body fat, cholesterol level, and overall fitness level.

The Park Avenue mind-set is goal oriented. Aim for 10,000 steps per day, about two miles. You may find that you are already taking 5,000 steps on an average day. If your long-term goal is 10,000 steps a day, just by walking your children to school and back, taking your dogs to the park, enjoying a stroll with a friend during your lunch hour, you can easily boost your number of total steps. Your pedometer will tell you exactly how many steps you have added. By keeping track of your progress, you will be encouraged and motivated to go the extra mile.

Alternatively, take an aerobics class or go bicycling; it doesn't really matter, but do this with purpose, and sweat! Swimming is not the best exercise for weight loss and does not increase bone mass, but it is a good exercise for strengthening the body and improving respiratory capacity.

No Time for Daily Exercise?
This is the most common excuse I hear when I recommend increasing your activity level. On a personal note, as a medical intern and as a resident I put in extremely long hours at the hospital; but instead of going home after a 24- or 36-hour shift, I went to the gym. I ran on the treadmill or took a class, and it energized me. I then showered, went home, and slept like a baby. I certainly didn't feel like doing this many a time,

but that is what makes the difference. If you only do it when you feel like it, it won't work!

Day 1 Menu

BREAKFAST:
Two scrambled omega-3 eggs with 1 ounce of low-fat cheese (such as Alpine Lace low-fat Swiss, Jarlsberg Lite, or part-skim mozzarella) and the fresh herbs of your choice: parsley, tarragon, chives, etc.
One-half cup of berries. Blueberries are very high in antioxidant vitamins; strawberries give you more vitamin C than orange juice. Note: One-half cup is equal to 2 handfuls of blueberries or 5 sliced medium-size strawberries.
Coffee or tea, with skim milk if desired
Calcium = 150 mg

MIDMORNING:
A cup of green tea. Also, drink several glasses of water throughout the morning.

LUNCH:
A large mesclun salad with 4 grilled large shrimp and balsamic vinaigrette or lemon juice
A large glass of mineral water*
1 cup of green tea
Calcium = 30 mg

AFTERNOON SNACK:
Caprese Salad (see page 183)
Drink several glasses of mineral water throughout the afternoon and have a cup of green tea.
Calcium = 300 mg

---

*All mineral waters are not created equal. The calcium content varies widely by brand. My favorite is San Pellegrino and I have it delivered by the case. It has a gentle carbonation and a high calcium content, 120 mg per liter. Bubbles are also filling and add a festive air. Serve it in a Baccarat champagne flute and think of it as your healthy glass of Cristal!

DINNER:
A tossed mixed greens salad with 2 ounces of grated Parmesan cheese
    and balsamic vinegar or lemon juice
Red snapper (4 to 5 ounces) lightly brushed with olive oil and broiled
    or grilled
Steamed white asparagus spears with lemon zest
Dessert: 6 ounces of plain yogurt with cinnamon and Splenda, if
    desired
Calcium = 300 mg

BEDTIME:
Two calcium citrate with vitamin D supplements
Calcium = 600 mg
Absorbed calcium = 500 mg (remember, you can only absorb 500 mg)

Total daily calcium = 1,280 mg

Day 2 Menu

Drink a large glass of water and work out for one hour, upon rising.

BREAKFAST:
1 cup of plain yogurt and ½ cup of berries (choose fresh blueberries,
    strawberries, raspberries, blackberries, or a combination)
Coffee or tea, if desired
Calcium = 150 mg

MIDMORNING:
A cup of green tea. Also, drink several glasses of water throughout the
    morning.

LUNCH:
An egg-white omelet (3 to 4 egg whites), with 1 ounce of feta cheese
    and red or yellow bell peppers or sliced shiitake or porcini
    mushrooms
A small green side salad with balsamic vinaigrette or lemon dressing
A large glass of mineral water
Calcium = 350 mg

AFTERNOON SNACK:
2 ounces of low-fat cheese with vegetables
Drink several glasses of mineral water throughout the afternoon and
    have a cup of green tea.
Calcium = 300 mg

DINNER:
Salade Niçoise with ½ cup of green beans, 6 kalamata olives, ¼
    teaspoon of capers, 4 anchovies, and 4 to 5 ounces of tuna, 1 hard-
    boiled omega-3 egg (eliminate the salad's traditional potatoes) with
    mustard vinaigrette or lemon juice. The total quantity of salad
    should be satisfying: Serve with 3 cups of romaine lettuce, torn into
    bite-size pieces.
A large glass of mineral water with a slice of lime or lemon
Dessert: 6 ounces of Fage Total 0 % yogurt with herbal tea
Calcium = 150 mg

BEDTIME:
Two calcium citrate with vitamin D supplements
Absorbed calcium = 500 mg

Total daily calcium = 1,450 mg

Salad Savoir Faire
A green salad can be a symbol of humdrum deprivation, or it can be
something that really pops on your plate. Learn not to think of salads as
just an obligation that you eat because you know you should. Salads can
be a delicious lunch or entrée, and the varieties are endless.

Salads don't have to be boring; it's not just about wilted Romaine lettuce smothered in dressing. Get creative with your greens. In choosing the
contents of your salad, make sure that they are of high quality. Tomatoes
that are out of season and have a rubbery texture will not give you pleasure. If tomatoes are out of season, substitute a vegetable that is in season.
How about a bright orange bell pepper or a fresh red-and-white-striped
radicchio? On the Upper East Side, we have plentiful markets that offer a
wide variety of gorgeous greens to choose from. Fresh Direct, whose white
and orange trucks can be found on every major thoroughfare around New

York, has an amazing selection of hearty organic greens. Whole Foods stores are popping up all across the U.S. with superb fresh vegetables.

The mix of gourmet salad greens called mesclun may include arugula, frisée, mâche, radicchio, dandelion greens, mizuna, oak leaf, and sorrel. Choose mesclun with crisp leaves and no signs of wilting. You can buy pre-mixed mesclun at any market today. It can be refrigerated in a plastic bag for up to 5 days. You can also make up your own by mixing and matching greens. Choose leaves that add interesting flavors, colors, and textures to the mix, such as endive, kale, escarole, swiss chard, or baby spinach.

Greens should be thoroughly washed and dried before being turned into salad, otherwise they will water down the dressing. Try using a salad spinner or, after shaking off most of the water, you can roll the washed greens in paper towels to help absorb the remaining moisture.

You can add all kinds of other vegetables to your salads depending on your mood. I generally prefer simpler salads that allow one or two ingredients to really shine, but to each his own. For a slightly sweet, mild anise flavor, add a chopped fresh fennel bulb. Cucumbers, red bell peppers, shredded cabbage, chopped celery, cauliflower, broccoli, and radishes add crunch. Lightly steamed asparagus or haricots verts that have been chilled can make great additions. Try roasting scallions, zucchini, yellow squash, or portobello mushrooms on the grill or roasting them in the oven before adding to salads, and serve chilled or slightly warm. Fresh pomegranate seeds add color and crunch and are very high in antioxidants.

To turn your salad into a satisfying meal, add grilled chicken, seafood, or tofu, or toss on some crumbled feta cheese or part-skim mozzarella, kalamata olives, or seeds.

Dressing It Up
Don't overdress your salad. You need just a small amount, about one teaspoon per person, if you toss well. In my plan, the salad itself is the main attraction, the dressing is just the finishing touch! A light, flavorful vinaigrette dressing (such as Ginger Soy or Lime-Shoyu, see page 188) will enhance the flavors of your salad instead of overpowering them.

Use a delicious balsamic vinegar, of which there is a wide range of variation in flavors. True balsamic vinegar is aged a minimum of six years and preferably twelve or more, and traditionally comes from Modena, a city in the Emilia-Romagna region of Italy. It is the unfermented juice of the white Trebbiano grape. The juice is boiled down to a sweet, intensely fruity syrup that is then aged in a series of barrels made from selected woods, including chestnut, mulberry, juniper, oak, and cherry, which gives it its dark color and pungent sweetness. Balsamic means "like balsam," referring to the fact that it is thick and aromatic. The finished vinegar is presented to the DOC, an overseeing body similar to those that govern the quality of French and Italian wines. Balsamic vinegars without this designation on the label are usually aged for six to twelve months in stainless-steel tanks, or aged for two to twelve years in wooden barrels. The finest quality is aged over 25 years and can cost $150 per bottle.

Select a cold-pressed extra-virgin olive oil—not the olive oil that you use for cooking. Salad olive oil should have a harvest date. The harvest date should be the current year, to ensure freshness. Try some of the wonderful green olive oils from Sicily that vary from region to region. The oils from the Mount Etna area have a rich, smoky flavor, and those grown on the coast surrounded by orange trees are somewhat fruity in taste! Explore different varieties and you will find new delights.

Day 3 Menu

Drink a large glass of water and work out for one hour, upon rising.

BREAKFAST:
1 cup calcium-enriched low-fat cottage cheese with ½ cup of berries
Coffee or tea, if desired.
Calcium = 300 mg

MIDMORNING
A cup of green tea. Also, drink several glasses of water throughout the morning.

LUNCH:
A large mesclun salad with radishes, tomato, and 4 ounces of canned sardines or Alaskan wild salmon (may be packed in oil, but be sure to drain this thoroughly), with vinaigrette or lemon juice dressing.
8 ounces of mineral water
Calcium = 50 mg

The addition of radish and tomato, with their red color, supplies lycopene. Studies have suggested that this antioxidant may lower the risk for prostate cancer and macular degeneration. Billy Baldwin, the legendary decorator, said that every room should have some red in it. From a nutrition point of view, every salad needs red, too!

AFTERNOON SNACK:
An 8-ounce container of plain 0% fat yogurt with cinnamon and
    Splenda, if desired
Drink several glasses of mineral water throughout the afternoon and
    have a cup of green tea
Calcium = 150 mg

DINNER:
Miso soup (see page 186)
Sashimi: 4 or 5 pieces of your choice, with low-sodium soy sauce
Decaffeinated green tea
Calcium = 100 mg

BEDTIME:
Two calcium citrate with vitamin D supplements
Calcium = 500 mg

Total daily calcium = 1,100 mg

Green tea has from early times been highly valued as a powerful medication. The Japanese custom of drinking green tea came from China in about A.D. 800. Buddhist monks, who had gone to China for study, returned to Japan bringing tea with them as a medicinal beverage. In recent years, research into the effects of green tea has made it increasingly clear that it has a place in preventing disease. Tea comes from the plant *Camillia sensis*. It is known to be rich in polyphenols, which are powerful antioxidants. Whether a tea is black, green, or white depends on the state of maturity at harvest. Black tea is mature tea that has fermented. Green tea is made from immature leaves containing a compound called epigallocatechin gallate, or EGCG, which protects the arteries against damage and may prevent cancer. It is one of the strongest antioxidants known. EGCG is only present in the green leaves and is oxidized as tea becomes mature and loses its green color. When the tea plant blooms, the blossoms themselves may be made into tea, which is called white tea.

Day 4 Menu

Drink a large glass of water and work out for one hour, upon rising.

BREAKFAST:
3 ounces of smoked salmon on ⅛ melon of your choice, with lemon and
    freshly ground pepper
Coffee or tea, if desired

MIDMORNING:
Drink several glasses of water throughout the morning.

> Smoked salmon and melon are a wonderful combination of tastes. It also may be served as a first course at a dinner party, providing a healthier alternative to prosciuto and melon. The melon may be cubed and wrapped with a small piece of salmon for a cocktail hors d'oeuvre. Talk about versatility!

LUNCH:
A large chopped salad (spinach, arugula, red and yellow bell peppers,
    radicchio, and red onion) with 4 to 5 ounces of grilled lean chicken,
    and balsamic vinaigrette or lemon juice
A large glass of mineral water
Calcium = 50 mg

AFTERNOON SNACK:
2 ounces of low-fat cheese with 1 cup of raw vegetables. (Remember the
    big glass bowl in the refrigerator with the colorful crudités? Open
    the door and have yourself a party!)
Drink several glasses of mineral water throughout the afternoon and
    have a cup of green tea.
Calcium = 300 mg

DINNER:
Tossed tricolor salad with arugula, endive, and radicchio, drizzled with
rosemary vinegar
Low-Fat Asparagus Cheese Soufflé (see page 203)
Calcium = 400 mg

BEDTIME:
Two calcium citrate with vitamin D supplements
Calcium = 500 mg

Total calcium = 1,250 mg

Day 5 Menu

Drink a large glass of water and work out for one hour upon rising.

BREAKFAST:
An omega-3 3-egg omelet with 1 ounce of low-fat cheese plus bell
peppers, mushrooms, and onions
Coffee or tea, if desired
Calcium = 150 mg

MIDMORNING:
A cup of green tea. Also, drink several glasses of water throughout the
morning.

LUNCH:
4 ounces of grilled red snapper, with a side salad
Large glass of mineral water
Calcium = 50 mg

AFTERNOON SNACK:
8 ounces of low-fat plain yogurt with cinnamon and Splenda, if desired
Drink several glasses of mineral water throughout the afternoon, and
have a cup of green tea.
Calcium = 150 mg

DINNER:
4 to 5 ounces grilled wild Alaskan salmon or Arctic char, lightly
   brushed with olive oil
Lightly steamed asparagus spears with lemon juice with freshly ground
   pepper
Steamed broccoli topped with 1 ounce of grated Parmesan cheese
A glass of skim milk
Calcium = 400 mg

BEDTIME:
2 calcium citrate with vitamin D supplements
Calcium = 500 mg

Total calcium = 1,250 mg

Arctic char resembles salmon in its bright orange-pink color and appearance, but is genetically more closely linked to trout. When grilled, the skin is crisp and dark brown due to its high fat content, and it can also be smoked. This species is usually quite expensive and is most often found in upscale restaurants.

Amber, one of my single patients in her thirties, was on a date at one of New York's classically romantic restaurants, Café des Artistes. She was en route to the powder room as she gave her date the liberty of ordering for her, giving him just the guideline of, "I'd like a nice piece of fish; you can choose for me." When the entrées arrived, she was served a deep orange piece of what she quite naturally mistook for grilled salmon. Eager to please the dapper investment banker sitting across from her, she complimented him on his excellent choice. Her date, who fancied himself to be quite a New York foodie, exclaimed with disdain, "My dear girl, that's a rare wild Arctic char, not salmon!" Amber was mortified, and for the rest of the evening said very little to avoid making any other faux pas. Funnily enough, she ended up dating that banker for a while, and they shared a few good laughs about that incident together.

Day 6 Menu

Drink a large glass of water and work out for one hour, upon rising.

BREAKFAST:
8 ounces of low-fat plain yogurt and ¼ cup of berries
Coffee or tea, if desired
Calcium = 150 mg

MIDMORNING:
A cup of green tea. Also, drink several glasses of water throughout the
    morning.

LUNCH:
1 cup of low-fat calcium-enriched cottage cheese and a side salad; for
    example, 3 cups of mesclun with balsamic vinegar
Mineral water
Calcium = 350 mg

AFTERNOON SNACK
2 ounces of Garlic Hummus (see page 191) with 1 cup of raw
    vegetables—use color as your guide: red, yellow, green, and orange
    bell peppers, carrots, zucchini, and cucumbers
Drink several glasses of mineral water throughout the afternoon, and
    have a cup of green tea.

DINNER:
A large spinach salad with sun-dried tomatoes and 5 large grilled
    shrimp (lightly brush with olive oil for grilling) with balsamic vinegar
    or lemon juice
1 ounce of low-fat cheese
Mineral water
Calcium = 200 mg

BEDTIME:
2 calcium citrate with vitamin D supplements
Calcium = 500 mg

Total calcium = 1,200 mg

It was once thought that shrimp had no place in a heart-healthy diet because of their high amounts of cholesterol. It is now known that it is saturated fat that clogs arteries, not cholesterol. Five shrimp contain 50 mg of cholesterol and no saturated fat.

Sun-dried tomatoes are an Italian favorite. They are available in many forms. Avoid the oil-packed variety as these contain excessive calories. Purchase them dried and reconstitute by pouring boiling water over the tomatoes. Allow them to soak for five minutes. You have just saved yourself 100 calories!

Day 7 Menu

Take a day off from your workout and rest. Drink a large glass of water and do a good stretching routine of approximately fifteen minutes.

BREAKFAST:
1 cup of calcium-enriched cottage cheese and ⅙ of a melon (try
    honeydew, cantaloupe, casaba, or Crenshaw)
Coffee or tea, if desired
Calcium = 300 mg

MIDMORNING:
A cup of green tea. Also, drink several glasses of water throughout the
    morning.

LUNCH:
Grilled vegetables* (eggplant, fennel, yellow summer squash, and
    scallions) with 3 ounces of low-fat goat cheese, plus balsamic vinegar
    or lemon juice
Mineral water
Calcium = 350 mg

---

*Prior to grilling or broiling, paint the vegetables with the following mixture: 2 tablespoons of olive oil, ¼ cup of finely chopped fresh thyme, 1 or 2 cloves of finely chopped garlic. This recipe uses thyme but you can substitute any other herb that you enjoy.

AFTERNOON SNACK:
1 cup of low-fat plain yogurt with cinnamon and Splenda, if desired
Drink several glasses of mineral water throughout the afternoon, and
  have a cup of green tea.
Calcium = 150 mg

DINNER:
A tossed salad of ¼ pound of cremini or oyster mushrooms, 8 chopped
  walnut halves, and ½ head of Boston lettuce, with a dressing of 1
  tablespoon of walnut oil and 1 tablespoon of red wine vinegar
A 4-ounce grilled halibut steak with Carla's Salsa Verde (see page 187)
A glass of skim milk
Calcium = 300 mg

BEDTIME:
2 calcium citrate with vitamin D supplements
Calcium = 500 mg

Total calcium = 1,600 mg

This is the sample menu from week 1. Once you have completed the first week, you will be familiar with the plan and you should feel free to switch meals within the week; by this I mean have breakfast from day 1, lunch from day 7, a snack from day 3, and so on. Do not change the basic meals, as these are the foods that you should eat every day for phase 1. You have undoubtedly noticed that there is protein at every meal and snack. Studies have shown that the energy of metabolizing protein is greater than the energy cost of metabolizing carbohydrates; this translates into an efficient way to lose weight and to maintain lean muscle. Eat fruit only in the morning. You need high-quality protein and vegetables, and 1,200 mg of calcium daily.

While I have advised fish only for the first week, it is not as limiting as it seems, as fish is a broad category. Salmon is completely different from red snapper, which is completely different from lobster, taste-wise. I suggest that you keep it interesting by consuming a large variety of fish. And, as I mentioned earlier, you are free to substitute skinless chicken or turkey.

WHAT ABOUT MERCURY POISONING FROM FISH?

Mercury in our oceans and streams comes primarily from coal-fired power plants, which release mercury into the air. Rain causes these emissions to fall into our waters, where the mercury becomes concentrated within the bodies of the fish. Shellfish are somewhat protected, and smaller fish, such as anchovies or sardines, do not accumulate a large amount because of their size. Because larger fish eat the small fish, mercury builds up in their bodies. Long-lived large fish have the greatest exposure. The FDA warns us to avoid swordfish, king mackerel, tilefish, and shark.

The danger of mercury is to the developing nervous system. Women who are pregnant or want to become pregnant, and children, are advised to avoid the above fish. Children should not be given canned tuna on a regular basis but, sad to say, it is a staple in many children's lunch boxes. For men, and for women who are not concerned with pregnancy, there has been some suggestion that high mercury levels may nonetheless cause cardiovascular disease. So it is best for everybody to avoid fish with a high mercury content. (See pages 232–38 for a list of the FDA mercury content of seafood.)

I have explained the benefits of fish's omega-3 fats. Populations with a low incidence of cardiac disease are the populations that eat the most fish. Alaskan wild salmon, high in omega-3, is a wonderful addition to your diet. Alaskan waters are pure and the salmon live for only one year; thus the mercury content is minimal.

Recent media reports have related that some fish, including farmed (not wild) salmon, contain toxic substances called PCBs. Polychlorinated biphenyls, PCBs are mixtures of up to 209 individual chlorinated compounds (known as congeners). Fish can absorb PCBs from contaminated sediments and from their food. Studies have found that the fishmeal fed to farmed salmon is highly contaminated with PCBs. Farmed salmon are fatter and generally bigger in size and contain more fat than wild salmon.

PCBs are stored in fat cells and remain there for an extended period of time. Wild salmon does not contain PCBs. Buy your salmon from grocers or fishmongers who can guarantee the source of their produce; be aware that some unscrupulous restaurants and grocers mislabel farmed salmon and sell it at a higher price as wild salmon.

How Much Weight Can I Lose in Two Weeks?

Often diets promise unrealistic or unhealthy weight loss. Besides being untruthful, this is a disservice to people following the plan. If dieters do not achieve the magical promised number they are disappointed, believing they and/or the diet has failed. These negative feelings are a key reason for giving up on a diet. They have no place in this plan!

I'll give it to you straight, without any hype:

- How much you will lose depends upon how overweight you are. The higher your initial weight, the higher your initial weight loss. So if you are only 10 pounds overweight, do not expect to lose it all in two weeks. Allow yourself three weeks or a month. The time will pass quickly and you will lock into a new, health-promoting eating style during that time. Keep your goal in mind and stay focused.
- Men often lose weight faster than women, because their greater muscle mass enables them to burn more calories.
- Much of the weight lost initially on any diet is water weight. In the case of alcohol indulgence or excessive carbohydrate intake, this can be as much as 7 to 10 pounds of water weight in the first week! After the first week, a weight loss of 1 to 2 pounds per week is the medical ideal. To reach your weight-loss goal, stick to the plan: Exercise for one hour daily, maximize calcium intake, control portion size, include high-quality protein in every meal, and eliminate processed foods and simple carbohydrates.
- If you are adhering to my plan carefully, measuring portion sizes and exercising daily yet do not lose at least 2 to 4 pounds during the first week or two, then there is a high probability that you have a metabolic problem. You should consult a physician and have your metabolism evaluated. Your thyroid may be underactive, or

you may have type 2 diabetes—both of these conditions can go unrecognized and cause weight gain.

- Continue phase 1 until you are close to your goal: within 5 pounds if you are a woman, or 7 pounds if you are a man.
- This plan is all about health. Phase 1 will take off those extra pounds. Phase 2 will keep them off.

Phase 2

By now you should be near your goal weight. Congratulations! A wonderful change has occurred with your body and mind. You have said yes to life. You have conquered cravings and hunger, and achieved a healthy weight. While there are others who are stuck in the rut of *"I only wish I could . . . ,"* you have realized within yourself the ability to change, and your own power over your destiny. This is strong stuff and it is real.

In phase 2, you will continue the health-promoting eating style that you began in phase 1. But first, take stock of how far you have come. How many sizes and inches have you lost, how good do you feel when you move, and how much lighter do you feel?

Stand in front of a full-length mirror and appraise your body. Notice how the belly fat has melted away, how your thighs no longer overlap, how well-defined is your muscle mass. You may not look like the latest super-model or the governor of California, but you are magnificent in your own way. Take a moment to congratulate yourself on this! It is appropriate for you to be proud of your accomplishment. This wonderful change is due to proactive behavior on your part. It took perseverance and self-discipline.

> *Losing weight is 90 percent mental. It is the mind-set of goal-directed behavior.*

Make a pledge to yourself to maintain this way of life, for your health.

YOUR GOOD-HEALTH PLEDGE

1. I will be thankful for every day and continue to live in a health-promoting manner.
2. I will prevent myself from becoming overly hungry by consuming protein-rich snacks, not carbohydrate-rich snacks.
3. I will anticipate hunger by keeping healthy snacks available.
4. I will continue to maintain a high calcium intake because of its numerous health benefits to my body.
5. Every day, I will give my body the exercise that it requires. I realize that 30 minutes to 1 hour is a small portion of my day and is an investment in my health.
6. I will not eat processed foods.
7. I will drink water throughout the day.

The goal of phase 2 is to gradually introduce foods that were restricted during phase 1. In phase 1, your plate was limited, to promote optimal weight loss. Phase 1 provided your body with everything it needed nutritionally but without the extra calories. If there you had a carbohydrate addiction, phase 1 eliminated it. Phase 1 set new patterns that you should continue for life, such as getting rid of empty calories in the form of processed foods, exercising daily, and being mindful of the nutritional value of each food that you consume. But even the most dedicated dieter will desire variety after a few weeks. Phase 2 provides additional food choices and serves as a transition to a lifetime of healthy eating. This plan is for life. Sure, you will have an occasional lapse—after all, you are only human—but if you are on the health track for 90 percent of the time, a small slip won't make a difference. Phase 2 is designed to allow you to continue to lose weight while adding more food until reaching maintenance level.

During phase 2, eat the breakfasts recommended in phase 1. It is important to begin every day with protein; by doing so, you will curb hunger. Studies show that people who start their day with a protein breakfast are less hungry during the morning, consume less food at lunch, and are more likely to maintain a slim body. Make sure to drink water throughout the day; 2 to 3 liters (quarts) is your daily goal. Save your snacks for the afternoon, as you learned in phase 1.

Week 1

For a protein source, you may substitute 4 ounces of grilled or roasted organic chicken or turkey or meat for the fish, to add variety to your meals. Vary your meals by having fish one day and chicken or turkey the next. You may vary the preparation by making kabobs with bell peppers and tomatoes and chicken. You will still lose weight on the program.

LUNCH:
Grilled chicken Caesar salad (4 ounces of grilled chicken, served over romaine lettuce with 1 ounce of Parmesan cheese), with mustard vinaigrette served on the side and lightly drizzled over salad
A large glass of mineral water with lemon or lime

OR

A 4-ounce grilled turkey burger over tricolor salad with balsamic vinaigrette served on the side and lightly drizzled over the burger
Large glass of mineral water with lemon or lime

DINNER:
Swifty's on Lexington Avenue serves one of my favorite dishes:
First course: Tuna carpaccio (2 ounces of fresh tuna, flattened so it fills the plate and "fools the eye" that you are eating a larger amount of food) served with ginger, green onions, and capers
Main course: Chicken paillard (4 ounces) with grilled seasonal vegetables
A large glass of mineral water with lemon or lime

OR

First course: Ice-cold gazpacho
Main course: Roasted turkey breast (4 ounces) with steamed spinach
   and one-half a roasted tomato, topped with olive oil and Parmesan
   cheese
Mineral water

When it comes to turkey, either light or dark meat is fine; just watch your portion size. Portions should be 4 or 5 ounces; this is the size of your palm plus one-third the length of your fingers, or roughly the size of a Palm Pilot. Controlling portion size is vital to maintaining a healthy weight. Even healthful foods will cause weight gain when eaten in excess.

Turkey burgers served in restaurants often have the skin included in the ground meat. This can result in their having as much saturated fat as a hamburger. If you want a turkey burger, go to an excellent butcher shop such as Lobel's or Leonard's on the Upper East Side, and have skinless turkey ground while you wait. In other parts of the country, rely on the best butcher shop you can find or visit Whole Foods.

If you enjoy lean red meat, you may add this back into your diet. Are you missing red meat now? I prefer to eat organic meat. Beef, lamb, pork, and venison are all acceptable. Consume small quantities and trim away all visible fat. The American Heart Association suggests that red meat be consumed no more than twice per week. Be aware that the standard size for most fillets is 8 ounces, so slice a filet in half at the start of your meal and consume only that amount at one sitting.

> *Portion control is an essential element of my diet plan. In a restaurant, you will almost always be served more food than you should eat.*

Joshua, a corporate attorney, entertains his clients at clubby, beefy hot spots like the Palm, the Post House, and Sparks Steakhouse (famous for having been the site of the murder of Paul Castellano by John Gotti, which is attributed to his rise to fame in organized crime). The size of Sparks's dining room is second only to the enormous size of the portions they serve. They actually have live lobsters on the menu from 3 pounds all the way up to 5¾ pounds! The restaurant prides itself on their "extra thick" rib lamb chops, a heaping plate of three large slabs of lamb, which Joshua has a particular weakness for. After working with him, I suggested that he order his favorite lamb chops, but ask for only one to be served to him, and give the other two chops to his driver to dig into. In this way, Joshua could satisfy his love for a great grilled lamb chop, stick on his meal plan, and make his driver very happy all in one go. Since he is a frequent patron of Sparks and often has a table reserved, the waiters know in advance to do the portion control for him, and Johnny, his longtime driver, knows to pick up the leftovers every time he brings Joshua there to dine.

HETEROCYCLIC AMINES

When meat (beef, pork, fowl, and fish) is cooked at high temperature, chemicals form that are not present in the uncooked meat. One of these chemicals, heterocyclic amines, may increase cancer risk. Temperature is the key feature in the formation of heterocyclic amines. Barbecuing, broiling, and frying produce the largest amounts of heterocyclic amines because the meats are cooked at very high temperatures. Cut off any burned portion of the meat!

FAST FOOD

The next time you pass a fast-food restaurant and get a whiff of the animal fat they use to fry potatoes, chicken, and fatty beef, think of a scene out of *Supersize Me*. That should zap any possible cravings you might have. There is a McDonald's on Third Avenue at Eighty-fifth Street, where the nannies park their carriages outside and congregate. I often wonder if some of my patients know that their pedigreed children are being fed McNuggets, Big Macs, and Happy Meals every day. It is called fast food because they serve it quickly—but it sticks fast to your arteries for a very long time!

On the Upper East Side, we have a healthy fast-food chain of cafés with a bright orange logo, called Better Burger (www.better burgernyc.com). They serve ostrich, tuna, soy, chicken, and turkey burgers. They call these "better burgers" because they are made from antibiotic- and hormone-free meat and poultry. Hale and Hearty Soups is another small restaurant that serves home-made soup and salads.

Week 2

The next item that should be added back to your diet is fruit. Fruit was only included at breakfast in phase 1, so how about adding an additional piece of fruit as part of your afternoon snack, in addition to the cheese or yogurt that you are already eating then. Do not eliminate the protein/calcium portion of your afternoon snack; eat 1 piece of fruit with it.

Apples or pears are equivalent in calories and fiber, so I suggest that these be your first choices. Both of these fruits are a tasty complement to cheese. With yogurt, you might add ½ cup of berries or a sliced peach. Melon is particularly good with 1 cup of low-fat cottage cheese— you may add ⅛ of any type of melon you enjoy. During summer, you may eat any delicious fruit that is in season; just watch your portion size—

remember, only one piece of fruit combined with protein. Steer clear of bananas, as they are high on the glycemic index. (The glycemic index is a measurement of how much a particular food will cause blood glucose to rise. Bananas are near the top of the list.)

SNACK:

1 medium-size apple or pear with 2 ounces of low-fat cheese

A glass of mineral water or a cup of green tea

If you are on the road, this snack travels exceptionally well, especially Bonbel Mini Light cheese. This semisoft cheese is coated with paraffin, so it will be fine without refrigeration during the day. It has a mild flavor and buttery texture, and is a delicious accompaniment to fruit.

OR

1 6-ounce container of Fage Total 0% yogurt with 1 peach or plum or ¼ cup of papaya or mango. These summer fruits are only available for a short time; enjoy them as a seasonal treat.

A cup of green tea or a large glass of mineral water

OR

In winter, try a baked Rome apple with cinnamon and 2 ounces of Vermont light Cheddar cheese. The baked apple is exceptionally filling.

A cup of green tea

OR

½ cup of low-fat cottage cheese with 1 medium-size orange or 2 nectarines

A large glass of water or a cup of green tea

OR

A mini smoothie made with a 6-ounce container of Fage Total 0% fat yogurt and ¼ cup of blueberries, 2 medium-size strawberries, 1 kiwi, and 3 ice cubes

A cup of green tea

Again, as you progress to adding a piece of fruit in the afternoon, re-member to always include protein and calcium. Each of the above snacks will provide protein, calcium, and—from the fruit—antioxidants to help you build and repair your body. You will feel satisfied and continue to lose weight. But even more important, you have broken away from reach-ing for the sugary snacks of weight gain and poor health that were doing nothing but harm to your body.

Week 3

At this point, you will be selecting from fish, poultry, and meat en-trées at lunch and dinner, in addition to consuming a wide variety of veg-etables. You will now be having two pieces of fruit per day: one with breakfast and one with your afternoon snack. It is perfectly fine to con-tinue along with this plan, or, if you like, you may now include legumes in your meal plan. Legumes are dried beans and are a good protein source, are high in fiber and rich in omega-3 fat, and provide a wonderful lunch in the form of soup. Legumes include lentils, black beans, navy beans, black-eyed peas, and cannellini. For lunch this week, include an 8-ounce serving of bean soup, with a side salad of mixed green vegetables and a balsamic vinaigrette. Avoid bean soups containing potato or rice, for now. Legumes are somewhat starchy, and the addition of potato or rice will be pushing the starch envelope! The soup may contain other vegeta-bles, such as onions, carrots, spinach, asparagus, or broccoli. If you pre-pare soup on the weekend and freeze it in 8-ounce containers, you will have a hearty and readily available lunch.

LUNCH:
8 ounces of black bean soup topped with 1 ounce of low-fat Cheddar cheese
2 cups of mixed greens salad with balsamic vinaigrette
A large glass of mineral water

OR

8 ounces of white bean and escarole soup
3-egg-white omelet with 1 ounce of Swiss cheese and diced tomatoes
A large glass of mineral water with lemon or lime

DINNER:

4 to 5 ounces of grilled cod, served over ½ cup black-eyed peas, with 1
     cup of steamed collard greens or spinach
A large glass of mineral water with lemon or lime

OR

5 grilled medium-size shrimp over ½ cup of red lentils, with 1 cup of
     steamed broccoli
A large glass of mineral water with lemon or lime

In New York City there are a number of restaurants that specialize in
soup. Among the best is Hale and Hearty Soups, which has several
branches throughout the city, including one on Lexington Avenue and
Seventy-eighth Street. All their soups are made fresh daily and are listed
as vegetarian, low fat, and dairy free, when applicable. The restaurant
also has soups with shrimp, beef, chicken, or turkey. One of my favorites
is the Spiced Lentil with Spinach Soup.

Week 4

You may now include sweet potatoes. That might seem like a strange
choice, because thus far the plan has been quite low on starchy foods. We
are adding sweet potatoes because they are high in vitamins, notably
beta-carotene, and also in minerals (potassium and calcium). You may
add one-half baked sweet potato two to three times per week. Sweet potatoes are not really part of the potato family; continue to avoid regular
(white) potatoes. Like white bread and white rice, white potatoes are
simple starches with little fiber, and have a tendency to stimulate
overeating.

*Do you know that the longest-lived people on earth, the Oki-
nawans, have a diet that includes high amounts of sweet potatoes?*

Week 5

Nuts may now be included in your diet. Nuts are often thought of as unfriendly to weight loss. But in fact, if you manage portion sizes and don't overconsume them, nuts are satiating and can help you to avoid feeling deprived. Nuts are actually seeds that are covered with a hard shell. They are a good source of protein, fiber, vitamins A and E, calcium, phosphorus, potassium, and healthy (monounsaturated) fat. Just limit your portion size because they are high in carbohydrates, oils, and calories. Avoid nuts packed with salt or in oil. Macadamia and Brazil nuts are particularly high in fat content and calories.

AFTERNOON SNACK:
1 cup of fat-free plain yogurt with ¼ cup of berries and 4 chopped
  walnuts. (You will get 15 g of protein from the yogurt, and 4 g of
  protein from the walnuts.)
2 ounces of Parmesan cheese with 10 almonds

DINNER OR LUNCH:
Top your salad or vegetable with a handful of almonds or other nuts of
  your choice.

NUTS AND SEEDS

Here is how 1 ounce of nuts stack up nutritionally:

Almonds. Twenty-two whole almonds have 170 calories. They
  are high in fiber and protein, have more calcium than
  any other nut, and are a good source of vitamin E, iron,
  magnesium, and have 9 g of monounsaturated fat. In addition, they are rich in the amino acid arginine, which affects
  the body's production of nitric oxide, which relaxes blood
  vessels.

(continued)

Walnuts. Fourteen walnut halves have 185 calories. The important nutritional benefit of walnuts is that they are high in arginine and in alpha-linolenic acid, which converts within the body to an omega-3 fat.

Cashews. Eighteen cashews have 165 calories. Although high in saturated fats, cashews also have a fair amount of monounsaturated fats.

Hazelnuts. Twenty hazelnuts have 178 calories. They are an excellent source of magnesium, phosphorus, potassium, and thiamin, also a good source of vitamin E. They are high in monounsaturated fats.

Peanuts. Thirty-three peanuts have 165 calories. Actually legumes, not nuts, they have high levels of arginine, are high in protein, and are an excellent source of magnesium, niacin, and folate. They have a fair amount of monounsaturated fat.

Seeds are nutritious and crunchy, as a snack or added to other foods.

Pumpkin Seeds. Can be eaten cooked (see page 217). Delicious toasted and sprinkled, while hot, with low-sodium soy sauce and served on salads. They are rich in protein, iron, zinc, and phosphorus. Three and a half ounces (100 g) of pumpkin seeds contain 29 g of protein, 11.2 mg of iron and 1,144 mg of phosphorus.

Sesame Seeds. A good source of protein and calcium, 100 g of sesame seeds contain 26.4 g of protein, 12.6 mg of vitamin B_3, 7.8 mg of iron, 131 mg of calcium, and 10.3 mg of zinc.

Sunflower Seeds. The seeds can be eaten whole from the shell, raw or cooked. They can be added to breads and cakes, or sprinkled over salads or breakfast cereals. A good source of potassium and phosphorus, 100 g of sunflower seeds also contain 24 g of protein, 7.1 mg of iron, and 120 mg of calcium.

Week 6

Complex carbohydrates, such as whole-grain bread and cooked whole grains, may be included into your diet plan now. Indulge in these two to three times per week. Do not have both on the same day or on the day that you have legumes or a sweet potato, or you may stop losing weight. Be very careful with this. The serving size is of utmost importance: One serving is ½ cup of cooked grains (such as brown rice) or one slice of whole-grain bread. If you find that eating so many carbohydrates stimulates your hunger, eliminate them.

When you reach your goal weight, you can add cereal. Eating carbohydrates early in the day has been found to slow weight loss, whereas eating protein promotes weight loss. It is like a resetting of the metabolism, with protein turning the volume up and carbohydrates turning it down. If you must have cereal, make sure that it is one with added protein. The correct serving size is 1 cup. On a cold winter day hot oatmeal just seems right! Make full-bodied slow-cooked oatmeal, as opposed to the packaged kind where you stir in hot water.

While skim milk is a great accompaniment to cereal, for variety try low-fat yogurt—either of these will add more protein. Make sure that your cereal has at least 5 g of fiber. I would not suggest having cereal as a snack, particularly in the evening. This is how many people slip back into the high-carbohydrate diet. If you consume cereal, make sure it is only 1 cup and only for breakfast, no exceptions.

GREAT GRAINS

Whole-grain foods are richer in fiber. Look for the word "whole" in front of the grains used on the label, to be sure they haven't been processed. Grains are really seeds that are made up of bran, which is the outer shell, endosperm, and the germ. The bran contains fiber, B vitamins, and trace minerals. When

(continued)

adding whole grains to the diet in the form of breads or cereals, always consider their fiber content. If a slice of bread doesn't provide at least 3 g of fiber, pass it by for one that does.

One great-tasting high-fiber bread is Mestemacher. This has 5 to 6 g per slice and comes in a variety of whole grains, including rye with muesli, whole rye, sunflower bread, three-grain, and fitness bread. Other brands that have high fiber counts include the Organic Baker and Ezekiel. If you like wraps, Damascus Bakery (www.damascusbakery.com) makes Flax Roll Ups that are made from organic flax flour. These are a good source of omega-3, and each roll up has 9 g of dietary fiber.

Cereals can be a fiber source also, but should only be eaten in moderation. The best choices, such as All Bran, have 5 g or more per serving. Kashi Go Lean has 8 g per serving (www.kashi.com). Just a 1-cup serving supplies 40 percent of your daily fiber needs and 20 percent of your daily protein needs.

Oatmeal is an old favorite. The best is McCann's Slow-Cooked Irish Oatmeal because of its high fiber content—4 g per $1/2$-cup serving. "Steel-cut" refers to the process of cutting the hulled oat into approximately four small pieces; rolled oats are steamed and pressed through rollers. Steel-cut oats have slightly more fiber and a chewier texture. Instant oatmeal is not a good choice because of its lower fiber content. When buying cereal, always check the label for its fiber content.

What About Wine?

Populations that consume wine with meals have a lower risk for cardiovascular disease. The amount of wine with associated health benefits is two glasses (or 7 ounces of wine) for a male and 1 glass (or $3^{1}/_{2}$ ounces of wine) for a female. The recommendation given is for 6-ounce wineglasses not filled to the brim. Unfortunately, just as portions have grown with food servings, wineglasses are bigger, too. Tiffany's top-selling wineglass is their 15-ounce crystal multipurpose wineglass. The "Claro" wineglass from Pottery Barn holds 16 ounces. While it is true that the larger size glass will allow wine to "breathe" more, there will also be additional wine poured into the glass. It is easy to see how you could end up unwittingly drinking far more than the recommended amount. Also, in restaurants and at dinner parties, wineglasses are refilled often without the diner being aware of it. So just be aware of how much wine you are actually consuming.

If you enjoy drinking wine, add it after you are comfortably at your goal weight. It is best if you introduce alcohol gradually by alternating a glass of wine with a glass of water or by having a wine spritzer. Just as you had a plan with everything else, you must have a plan with alcohol. Decide how many drinks you will have per week. Make this decision in advance, so that you are not caught up in the moment and end up just doing what everyone else is doing. Whatever you decide, stick with it. My suggestion is one to two glasses of wine per week, as this amount doesn't seem to cause weight gain.

One of the big issues for my very social patients is how to avoid alcohol at a party, gala, wedding, or the country club. At a party, the technique is to hold a glass of anything in your hand. At least at the beginning of the plan, I recommend that my patients order a club soda or mineral water with lime so they don't feel self-conscious while everyone is drinking around them.

Men have long known that women become intoxicated on a smaller amount of alcohol.

Women generally weigh less than men, so the same amount of alcohol becomes more concentrated in a smaller body mass. Women process alcohol less efficiently. Studies show that women produce less of a stomach enzyme called alcohol dehydrogenase, which breaks down alcohol before it enters the blood; alcohol dehydrogenase is about 58 percent less efficient in females. Therefore, women become intoxicated far more easily than men.

One of my young patients, Julianna, keeps an immaculate journal. She writes down everything she consumes in great detail, highlighting any transgressions in yellow. She keeps her food diary right in her wallet so she can take it everywhere. She is very well organized and this accounts for a great deal of her success with my diet plan and in her profession. I am very proud of her. One of her journal entries caught my attention. In yellow she had highlighted ONE MARTINI. I asked her what happened. She told me she had gone to the King Cole Bar at the St. Regis Hotel on East Fifty-fifth Street. The King Cole Bar is famous for its beautiful Maxfield Parrish mural and for being the birthplace of the Red Snapper Cocktail, now commonly known as the Bloody Mary. Julianna said the bar makes the best martinis, but they are really expensive, about $18. As soon as she left my office, I called the King Cole Bar to find out what made these martinis so wonderful. I asked them what they put in their martinis, and the bartender read off the usual list of ingredients; gin and dry vermouth. So I asked him, "Then why are they so expensive?" He answered, "Because we give you twice as much, lady." That explained Julianna's slip; she thought she was having one martini but it was really the equivalent of two.

Think of it this way: alcohol = empty calories. It is also dehydrating and a depressant. Alcohol disrupts sleep and interacts with various medications. Wine has no protein or fat, but each 4-ounce serving contains between 2 and 6 carbohydrates and approximately 100 calories. Alcohol is tricky because it is so easy for it to get out of hand. It stimulates appetite, reduces inhibitions, and offers calories without satiety. It is true that after a stressful day, a glass of wine is relaxing, but this can quickly become a habit. Often people consume very high amounts of alcohol and may actually become dependent upon it without realizing it. We all have the potential for alcohol abuse.

HOW TO READ A LABEL

Label reading should be taught in school. Every man, woman, and child should learn to decode a food label. Just as you look at the price tag on anything you purchase, so should reviewing the label for nutritional content and ingredients be part of purchasing foods.

Know what is in the foods you are eating and don't rely on marketing slogans. Many of us are lured into believing that if a product is labeled "low-fat" or "low-carb" or "healthy," it must be good for you. I become immediately skeptical when I see these phrases on a product. They often use the color green because it is associated with natural, organics, and purity. Subliminal advertising ploys should set up red flags for you.

Nutritionally there are three key categories of any food:

- Carbohydrates
- Protein
- Fat

Nutritional claims made on the front of packaging are not enough to determine the actual contents of the product. If something has zero fat, then it must be either high protein or high carbohydrate. Most times, a fat-free processed product will have added sweeteners or salt, because fat makes food taste good and without it, manufacturers think the product needs extra flavoring. These sweeteners may be listed on the label in the form of sucrose, dextrose, glucose, high-fructose corn syrup, or malt. Salt may be disguised in terms containing "sodium." If you are going to choose a bar or snack to eat on the go, you need to know that many of these products marketed have just as many added sugars, if not more, than what we consider classic junk food.

Food manufacturers have overcomplicated the information on the label. Perhaps this is an attempt to keep us confused about what we are really eating. If you are too lazy or too busy to

(continued)

read labels, the one sure way to avoid choosing the wrong foods is to limit your selection to whole, pure, unprocessed foods! But it pays to become educated about the nutritional analysis of packaged foods, as some products may be good for you.

SAMPLE LABEL—WHAT YOU NEED TO FOCUS ON

NUTRITION FACTS:	AMOUNT/SERVING	%DV*
Serving size 1 bar (38 g)	**Total fat** 4 g	6%
Servings 1	**Sat. fat** 2.5 g	13%
Calories 150	Cholest. 1.5 mg	1%
Fat Calories 35	Sodium 125 mg	5%
	Potassium 35 mg	1%
Total Carb 19 g		6%
Dietary fiber 0 g		0%
Sugars 14 g		
Protein 10 g		
Vitamin A 0% Vitamin C 0%		
Calcium 6% Iron 10%		

*percent daily values based on a 2,000-calorie diet.

Focus on the **bold** items: serving size, servings, calories, total fat, saturated fat, dietary fiber, protein, and calcium. These are all that you need to be concerned with. Fat calories or the percentage of daily values for items are not important unless you are a nutritionist or if you have a rare metabolic problem.

Let's go through the important items one by one:

Servings. This tells you how many servings are present.

This is especially important for beverages. For example, a patient recently brought in a bottle of one of the trendy, colorful

(continued)

vitamin waters. What she had seen as 20 calories was revealed to be 20 calories per serving—and there were four servings in the bottle. There were 80 calories in a drink that she thought was just like water, and that she might have drunk in one sitting, not realizing the portion size. She could have had an apple or an egg for the same amount of calories, and it would have been much more satisfying.

Remember: Calories that you drink are far less satisfying than calories that you eat!

Serving size. This tells you what quantity is being described on the label—and does not usually represent the entire package or bottle.

Calories. This is where the fast-food industry (and "casual dining" restaurants) must step up to the plate and come clean. If people are aware of the real amount of calories in the foods they consume, at least they can make an informed decision as to whether to eat them or not.

Total fat and saturated fat. Both of these are important because saturated fat has been shown to elevate LDL, or "bad" cholesterol. It is recommended presently that levels of LDL cholesterol should be kept lower than 100 mg/dl. Therefore, the goal is to consume a low amount of saturated fat—not more than 3 g per serving of any one food.

Trans fats. These are even more harmful to the body. Trans fats are not required to be listed on labels at this writing. The reason for this is tremendous lobbying efforts by the food industry against including trans fats on food labels. In 2006, manufactur-

(continued)

ers will be required to list trans fats. Trans fats exist when a food contains partially hydrogenated vegetable oil. This is an ingredient of the vast majority of packaged baked goods, including cereals, cookies, and crackers. Check your pantry—you will be shocked! Mono- and polyunsaturated fats are the good fats; they lower the bad cholesterol. The prestigious Institute of Medicine has stated that there is *no* acceptable amount of trans fat allowed in the human diet. Look for packaged cereals and baked goods in health food stores, where the products may be safe. Even there, read your labels carefully.

Look for low amounts of saturated and trans fats.

Dietary fiber. The Institute of Medicine recommends 25 to 35 g of fiber per day. This is based on population studies that show a low risk for disease with this amount of fiber. Most Americans get about 10 g per day. Bread and cereals should be high fiber. Top sources are vegetables and fruits—not vegetable or fruit juice! Fiber lowers LDL cholesterol.

Protein. We need protein in our diets to build and repair tissue. Because you will be active and exercising daily, I recommend that you include protein with all meals. Make it a high-quality protein that is not high in saturated fat.

Calcium. This important mineral is vital for our health. It helps to preserve our bone health, keeps our blood pressure under control, and now it appears that it even helps with weight control.

Begin reading labels right away so that you know what you are putting in that magnificent body of yours.

Believe it or not, the nutritional data we just decoded was that

(continued)

of a "high-energy protein bar"! For the same amount of calories, you could have had a 6-ounce container of 0% fat yogurt with ¼ cup of fresh blueberries or raspberries, and 8 to 10 roasted chopped almonds as a topping (think of it as a healthy sundae!).

Now, let's look at the ingredients list on that same label:

Ingredients: High-fructose corn syrup, soy protein isolate, calcium caseinate, corn syrup, sugar, fractionated palm kernel oil, wheat flour, nonfat milk, lactose, cocoa (processed with alkali), natural flavor, oleic oil, sunflower oil, canola oil, soy lecithin, caramel color, dextrose, salt, sodium bicarbonate.

High energy? Yes, but this type of energy is not what you want. This will give you an energy spike and cause you to crash within an hour. Avoid anything that lists as its first ingredient "high-fructose corn syrup," "corn syrup," or sugar. Ingredients are listed in order of concentration, so if these are the first things listed that means that they are present in greater amounts than are the other ingredients. Palm oil is a tropical oil and one of the most highly saturated oils—a real artery-clogger!

FOODS TO AVOID

- ALL processed foods—packaged baked goods, sweets, snacks, meats—even "diet" cookies and crackers
- Anything with partially hydrogenated vegetable oil
- Dried fruit
- Fruit juice of any kind
- Soda—even diet soda
- Pretzels and crackers
- Frozen dinners

(continued)

The first two items contain oils that are harmful to the body. The other items are high in sugar. It is often thought that if something comes from fruit, it must be good for the body because fruits are natural, but nothing could be further from the truth! Fruit juices and dried fruits are sources of concentrated sugar, which spikes blood glucose and leaves you hungry. Fruit juices should be avoided because calories that you drink are less satisfying than calories that you eat. Dried fruits are "energy-dense" foods that pack high calories into a small volume. To maintain a healthy weight, you need the opposite: foods that are relatively low in calories with a large volume. So eat a piece of fresh fruit instead of dried fruit or a glass of fruit juice.

Carbonated beverages are a big source of calories for many people. Even diet soda, which may have no calories, contains preservatives, artificial colorings, sodium, and does not benefit the body. And its sweet taste reinforces the craving for sweets.

I believe Americans have a "sweeter palate" than other nations. When I prescribe a diet the most frequent questions I hear is, "Is it all right if I have diet soda?" or, "Is it all right if I have diet Jell-O?" "They don't have any calories." While it is true that these foods do not contain calories, what the person is really saying is, "I want something sweet." And if these diet foods are continued, the drive for sweetness is just positively reinforced.

This was recently shown in a very interesting study in laboratory mice. These mice were raised on a diet of artificially sweetened—no extra calories—mouse chow. There is a theory that all mammals have the ability to regulate their body weight. If you observe animals in the wild, they are just about the same weight—a herd of deer, a pride of lions, all members will be just around the same weight. This is also true for laboratory mice;

(continued)

they all weigh just about the same. Normal lab mice love sweet chow; when given a choice between sweetened mouse chow and regular mouse chow, they will go directly for the sweet chow . . . but then they will go back to the unsweetened chow. And, amazingly, they will also work out on the mouse treadmill to compensate for the extra calories. The mice naturally regulate their weight. But when the lab mice that had been *raised* on sweetened mouse chow were put into a cage with both regular chow and sweetened chow, they would consume only the sweet chow and they did not put in extra time on the mouse treadmill. They had, in effect, lost their natural ability to regulate their body weight! These mice had developed a strong preference for sweetness and they became quite fat. Overconsumption of non-calorically sweetened foods will cause you to build into your chemistry a drive for sweet tastes. While the diet foods themselves do not make you fat, they do cause you to crave sweet foods.

The lesson: Avoid simple carbohydrates, even those that seem unsweetened, as they will put the pounds back that you have worked so hard to get rid of and they will leave you hungrier than before. This means crackers and pretzels, too!

HOTEL SURVIVAL SKILLS

One of my clients called me because she was going to the New Orleans Jazz Festival. She sent me a list of the foods that would be available. Now, that was a challenge! There was not a lot for her to eat on the Bayou. Cajun or Creole cooking is a nutritionist's nightmare. It can be very rich, heavy, drenched in sauces and fat and sugar: po'boys, beignets, jambalaya, dirty rice. Alcohol is everywhere and people go there specifically to indulge. The best advice I could give her was to seek out the simplest grilled prawns and vegetables she could

(continued)

find, eat only tiny bites, and drink sparking mineral water with lime.

Traveling can really sabotage your healthy eating plan. Many of my clients are frequent flyers, and it is even harder to resist temptations when you are flying first class, living in airport executive lounges, and staying in four-star hotels. After a five-hour flight with a two-hour delay, you just want to take a hot shower, hit the mini bar, and crash. And most mini bars are loaded with sugary, high-carb snacks, chips, chocolate bars, and soda that will cost five bucks each. When you make your reservation, ask to have the mini bar removed, or refuse the key, or call the housekeeping service to empty it of all dangerous snacks. Request only mineral water and crudités. Stick with one hotel group as much as possible, and familiarize yourself with their room service menu. Better groups, such as Starwood Hotels that include the W, or the Ritz Carlton and Four Seasons, allow special meal requests that can be preordered. Just in case, you should always bring healthy travel snacks and beverages with you. It's all about planning.

OPTIMAL SNACK FOODS

- Nuts, such as almonds and walnuts (10 almonds have 85 calories, 7 walnuts have 185). Nuts are packed with nutrients, are good for your heart, and have a substance that helps lower blood pressure and even prevent diabetes. Yes, they contain fat but, hey, I think it's nuts not to eat them.
- Fat-free or low-fat yogurt (an 8-ounce container)
- Raw vegetables and fruit (1 cup of a medley of your favorite raw vegetables in a zip-top bag, plus an apple and 1 to 2 ounces of low-fat cheese is my recommendation for an airline travel pack)

(continued)

▼

- Low-fat cheese (1 to 2 ounces)
- Olives (try several varieties; 2 olives have approximately 10 calories)
- Hummus (¼ cup, freshly made, with 1 cup of vegetables)
- Blueberries. (Frozen, these are similar to a sorbet. A few will satisfy the craving for a sweet, and are rich in antioxidants. Or, if you are having fresh blueberries, enjoy ½-cup serving.)
- Boston Lite Popcorn, popped in canola oil (3 cups = 105 calories)
- Pumpkin seeds (¼ cup, roasted—see recipe, page 217)
- Fruit (1 piece, such as an apple or a handful of grapes or berries)
- Mineral water
- Teas of all kinds

All these foods provide nutritional benefits. Even popcorn is a good fiber source! Your goal for life is not to eliminate snacks but to consume only those that will nourish your glorious body.

Enjoying Your Veggies

With this program, the goal is to eat whole foods; that is, food as close to its natural state as possible. The more foods you eat that come straight from the garden, the better you are going to feel. If you live in an area where you can purchase good-quality, fresh, organically grown fruits and vegetables, this is ideal. If organically grown produce is not available, you can still reap many health and beauty benefits by eating conventionally grown produce. Vegetables should be bought as fresh and crisp as possible and kept in a cool, dark place to safeguard their vitamin content. They should never be soaked but washed and scrubbed thoroughly.

The nutritional content of healthy foods can be enhanced by careful cooking—or corrupted by overprocessing. Overcooked foods are missing some very vital elements needed by the body for its optimal functioning.

In general, vegetables should be crispy and not lose their color. Some cooking methods of even brief duration rob your food of vital vitamins. A classic example is the loss of vitamin C through boiling of vegetables. However, there are exceptions. In tomato paste, the beta-carotene actually becomes more concentrated as the tomatoes cook down, so this is actually a good source of that nutrient.

In America, we have on average only one vegetable serving per day, and it is usually a potato. We should try to consume nine or ten servings of nonstarchy vegetables per day. For maximum nutritional value, steam them in the microwave or on the stovetop with a small amount of water, or bring a pot of water to a rolling boil and rapidly cook the food. For example, spinach should be placed in boiling water for 15 seconds and then drained; put it in an ice-water bath or run it under cold water to stop the cooking process; it should be a deep, rich shade of vibrant green. Cooking softens plant fiber so that the vegetable is softer than if you would have it raw.

Steaming on the stovetop is easy. For best results, bring a small amount of water to a boil and use a two-piece steamer pot or a steamer itself. In case you don't know, a steamer is a small metal or bamboo basket that is placed over boiling water. When your vegetables are in the steamer they are not resting directly in the water. The pot should be covered. Steam has a higher temperature than water and cooks the vegetables more efficiently than does boiling them. The vegetables emerge brighter in color. Keep salt to a minimum (a pinch or two) during cooking, to draw out the flavor. Add herbs, spices, and garlic afterward instead of salt. You can save the extra liquid after cooking to use in soups.

Vegetables used in a salad should never be soaked. Wash them thoroughly in cold water and use a salad spinner to dry.

Healthy Salad Solutions

- Cold-pressed extra-virgin olive oil
- Canola oil
- Avocado oil
- Flaxseed oil
- Apple cider vinegar
- Red wine vinegar

- Balsamic vinegar
- Lemon juice

Feasting on Fruits

To protect their vitamin content, keep fresh fruits in the refrigerator or in a dark, cool place. They are apt to lose their vitamin content when left at room temperature. Possible exceptions would be fruits with heavy skin, such as bananas and pears. Citrus fruits should be refrigerated because the vitamin C will break down. As with vegetables, fruit should never be soaked but washed quickly in cold water. Trim as little as possible and never peel or cut until shortly before serving, to protect the vitamin C content. Because ripe, fresh fruits contain natural sugar, you don't need any additional sweetener.

Fresh, Frozen, or Canned?

Always choose fresh fruits and vegetables over canned varieties. Due to seasonal changes, sometimes we are not able to obtain fresh foods, so you may buy frozen whole foods. Avoid all frozen products that contain extra sauces, sweeteners, or chemicals. Flash freezing is a process where no sugar or preservatives are used. Read the label: It should just read "blueberries" instead of "blueberries, sugar, preservatives." One brand that carries pure organic frozen fruits, vegetables, and vegetable medleys is Cascadian Farm Organic (www.cascadian farm.com). For instance, they carry fresh, frozen whole-in-the-shell as well as shelled edamame, in case you have trouble locating these tasty soybeans in your local market. Also try their Harvest Berries, a medley of organically grown strawberries, blueberries, blackberries, and raspberries without added sugars or preservatives. Dark berries are super rich in antioxidants.

Food Do's and Don'ts

- Do buy the freshest foods available.
- Do buy the best-quality ingredients that you can find.

- Do get food home and into suitable storage conditions as quickly as possible.
- Don't overcook any food, especially vegetables and fruits.
- Don't undercook such foods as poultry, eggs, and meats as they are likely to be harboring bacteria, which are destroyed by heat.
- Don't refreeze foods that have already been frozen and defrosted.

Long-Term Maintenance, Wherever You Live

My plan is a plan for healthy eating all life long and can be followed by all who seek to reclaim vitality, regardless of where they reside. When you reach your goal weight you should be eating a wide variety of delicious foods that help you to stay slim and trim. I would like to emphasize that the plan is not about deprivation, but about *selectivity.* If you want to enjoy a special dessert, by all means, be my guest. You should have that dessert, but just not every night. And it should be really delicious, not just a store-bought sponge cake!

The people I see are mostly on the Upper East Side of Manhattan, but the principles of my plan can be adapted to any area. If your supermarket in Akron, Ohio, doesn't stock fresh arugula, then buy fresh spinach or a dark leaf lettuce. If you can't find Fage Total 0% yogurt in a supermarket in Lubbock, Texas, visit a health food store that has a selection of fat-free, unprocessed plain yogurts, or make your own. What this is about is approaching food in a manner that will benefit your health. Read labels. Be skeptical about health claims made for products. You have a responsibility to yourself to be aware of what it is that you are eating. In any city, in any country, you can refuse the bread basket. But if you want to have bread on occasion, it is OK. Is this a contradiction? Absolutely not. It just means that you are aware of the food you have chosen to consume and are not just eating out of habit or boredom. You eat a piece of bread because you have consciously decided to do so, and you don't do it all the time.

When you are at your goal weight, weigh yourself in the morning. By keeping track of your weight, it won't get out of control. If you find that you have gained a few pounds, address it right away. Go back to phase 1 for a week and the pounds will drop.

Chapter Five

CURB YOUR CRAVINGS:

THE STOP! WATCH! METHOD

Eat that you may live and not live to eat.
—ARISTOTLE

• • •

No matter how strongly motivated or self-disciplined you are while attempting to lose weight, inevitably there will come a time when you experience a craving. A craving has been defined as an intense desire for a substance. A smoker craves nicotine. A drug abuser craves cocaine or heroin. Food, too, may act like a drug, in that you may feel almost powerless to overcome the desire to eat something in particular, which is what differentiates a craving from hunger. The specificity of the craving is due to the fact that certain foods seem to stimulate certain neurotransmitters in the brain. Thus, the craving for chocolate stimulates serotonin, while fats are believed to be involved in dopamine release.

Cravings and Stress

Interestingly, cravings do not appear to be associated with one's degree of hunger. One may be hungry and yet not experience a craving. Hunger expresses a body's drive for food. A craving, however, is related to tension and mood. Giving in to cravings may be a technique we use to feel better during time of stress. Almost everyone can relate to this concept. Remember the time you were dumped by a lover or criticized unduly by a boss. What did you do? After wiping away your tears, you probably headed right for the Ben and Jerry's!

It is also interesting to note that one's response to a craving has different consequences for males and females in terms of whether the indulgence is perceived as helpful or not. Males do not experience negative feelings about themselves after giving in to a food craving whereas females report feelings of negative self-worth. No doubt this is due to the premium that society places on female attractiveness, as symbolized by a slim body. In essence, this is the scenario for women: Something upsets us, causing us to derive solace from a particular food, but after consuming the food we feel worse because not only does the original problem remain, but now we have guilt feelings over what we ate!

These negative feelings are particularly harmful when you are attempting to lose weight, because a small slip is often perceived by the dieter as confirmation of her worst fear: She just doesn't have the self-discipline that it takes to lose weight. This can become a self-fulfilling prophecy.

Surrendering to a craving can precipitate a binge-eating episode.

The mind rationalizes the scenario like this:

> My boss is so mean and hateful—she berated me in front of the entire office; I'm just going to stop at the bakery on the way home and pick up a half dozen (that's only six) of those cookies that I love. I'll eat one; what difference does one more make? I am going to just polish off the rest of the bag since I've blown my diet today anyway! Hey, I think the deli is still open—some ice cream will really top off those cookies! I feel like such a pig; I have no self-control. I can't even succeed at a stupid diet. I can't succeed at anything! I hate myself.

Alternatively, if you are able to get through a particularly stressful period without allowing food cravings to win, then a sense of mastery over food is achieved. When you are in control and have a sense of self-mastery, then you cope with any problem better. A food craving can actually be a helpful tool that can lead us to realization that we are able to control ourselves instead of leading us to negative feelings. The Stop! Watch! Method can help you to use these annoying cravings to your advantage.

Cravings and Time

Of course, food cravings are not always related to stress. They can occur at specific times of the day. They can be compared to your need for a morning cigarette, or for a cocktail as the clock strikes 6:00 P.M. You may want that blueberry muffin with your morning coffee, or a piece of pie in the afternoon, or a bowl of ice cream before bed. These eating patterns are simply habits that we need to change. They can be managed by just substituting a healthy alternative.

In my clinical practice, I advise my patients to keep a record of when their cravings occur. As simple as it may seem, if you keep this record you will find that your cravings are amazingly predictable. As a matter of fact, I am most susceptible to a craving at around 3:00 P.M. I can almost set my watch by it! For most people, the afternoon poses a problem with cravings. Other common problem times are just before and after dinner.

We plan so many aspects of our lives: what time we will arrive at work, what we will do on the weekends, how we will save our money, where we will go on our next vacation, and so on. Yet many neglect to plan for what to eat when hunger strikes. Because food is readily available, we don't concern ourselves with the details of what or how much we will consume. We simply reach for whatever is around that tastes good. These careless calories add up and slowly we put on more and more weight. A plan is needed for times of energy lag. First, determine when these times might occur. That they will occur is an absolute certainty.

Once you know the danger zones, you can prepare yourself by having a healthy snack at hand. If you don't plan ahead, you will leave yourself vulnerable to being at the mercy of the candy machine at work or eating whatever is in the fridge. In most cases you will find that, after having your snack, your craving has disappeared. Because time-centered cravings are so predictable, they are actually quite simple to control. The Stop! Watch! Method just quantifies their duration, adding another tool for control.

Mindless Eating

Mindless eating is what I refer to as the "couch potato syndrome." There are times when we are just plain bored. For some people, this boredom leads to eating. Hunger is not an issue here. In this instance food is a form of entertainment. Mindless eating can occur during long drives, on airplanes, at our desks at work during the day, and especially in front of the television. The calories from this eating style are not satisfying. Food consumption at mealtime is not reduced to adjust for these; often we even forget what we ate between meals. The answer is to have bottled water on hand so that you reach for that when you are bored.

Night Eating Syndrome

One type of time-centered craving that is troublesome is night eating. This syndrome is defined by skipping breakfast, consuming most of your calories during the late evening and at night, and chronic insomnia. It is during the insomnia period that people seek food; they typically consume simple carbohydrates during these episodes. Or they may readily fall asleep, yet awaken with an overwhelming desire to eat. The harmful eating style builds over the course of years and can be an extremely difficult pattern to break.

In an attempt to break the cycle, people may try taking a sleeping pill to overcome the night eating urge. This is not an effective solution. Usually what occurs is a breakthrough waking period so that they may eat and then fall asleep again. The end result is grogginess in the morning and a disruption of the sleep pattern. Plus, addiction is a real risk here. Over time you may become unable to sleep without pills, and a higher dose will be required to get the same effect. The normal rhythm of sleep is disturbed and extra weight can be gained from the stress put on the body!

How to Stop or Prevent Midnight Munching

Because this eating disorder is defined by skipping breakfast, the addition of a healthy morning meal is crucial in reversing the behavior. If you are consistently skipping breakfast and find that you are becoming a night owl who eats into the wee hours of the morning, you are putting yourself at risk for development of the night eating syndrome. So, begin your day with a protein-rich breakfast. Later, you can proceed to small meals spaced evenly throughout the day and include a calcium and protein snack before bed. Avoid simple carbohydrates and starches.

> *The perfect bedtime snacks are milk and a slice of turkey because they contain L-tryptophan, an amino acid that aids sleep.*

If you awaken, do not eat or drink anything other than water. With diligence this harmful cycle can be broken, and it is crucial that it be addressed, as it can lead to significant weight gain over time. Patients with this syndrome are frustrated by their weight gain since they eat so little during the day and can't quite grasp that the evening load of simple carbohydrates is responsible for both their weight gain and their continued insomnia! By eating the correct balance of complex carbohydrates and protein at appropriate intervals and adding physical exercise, they become slim and sleep through the night!

It is much easier to prevent this than to fix it after it develops. So get your eating and exercise plan on track now!

Break the Cravings Pattern with the Stop! Watch! Method

Once you have recognized that you have cravings and how they can sabotage your diet, it is time to get them under control. Time will be our ally in this task as we recognize the following simple fact: A craving generally lasts only 8 to 14 minutes.

Refusing to give in to a craving will feel somewhat uncomfortable but it will pass. We are not talking about days or hours, only minutes! You need to realize consciously that these few minutes can make the difference between success and failure on a diet. There is power in this knowledge because it allows us to take action to regain control. I have come up with a technique that I use in my clinical practice to help my patients gain control over their cravings.

First, identify the time of day that you are experiencing cravings. This will allow you to prepare for them by having a healthful snack at hand. Cravings are cyclical in nature. You may intuitively be aware of this hunger pattern but some people are not. I can almost guarantee that there will be a certain time of day when you are more vulnerable to allowing your appetite to go haywire but, if you identify this, you can control it.

The typical time span of most food cravings is 8 to 14 minutes. I know it feels longer, but as Einstein told us, "Time is relative." Knowing that a craving is limited in duration will give you the power to ride through it.

The Stop! Watch! Method

1. When a craving arises I ask my patients to set a stopwatch (which I provide) for fifteen minutes; during this time they are advised to drink a large glass of water and eat a protein snack. This allows their blood glucose to become normalized (if it had dropped) and, by "waiting out" the urge, they gain control. It sounds simple but it does work. We have all experienced this phenomenon: on the treadmill, when we want to stop with ten minutes to go and we just count down the minutes; when sitting in a boring lecture and we watch the minutes tick away until the time that the class is over; or even when we give children a "time out" when they are having a tantrum. All of these situations have the same idea: holding on until a specific amount of time elapses. A stopwatch quantifies the time that a craving lasts. And for a dieter to know that there are only a few minutes left is enormously helpful!

2. Drink a big glass of water. Because our brain may misinterpret the signal for thirst as a signal for hunger, drinking water eliminates unrecognized thirst from the picture. You may just be thirsty, so go for the water first. Drinking a glass of water is filling and good for you, too.

3. Have a protein snack. If the snack that you chose is in the form of a high-tryptophan source, which include turkey and dairy products, then so much the better. L-tryptophan is an amino acid that

is converted to serotonin, a neurotransmitter that impacts satiety, mood, and cravings. Recall how relaxed you feel after having turkey at Thanksgiving dinner, or how soundly you slept after having a glass of milk prior to retiring. These effects are due to the calming action of serotonin. There is a potent class of antidepressants that increases the amount of serotonin in the brain (serotonin reuptake inhibitors or SSRIs), and guess what they are used to treat? Binge-eating disorder! I am not implying that if you experience cravings you will develop, or you have, a binge-eating disorder. Binge eating is a recognized psychiatric diagnosis whereby an individual experiences a loss of control and consumes far more than a normal individual would eat within a given period of time. But it is interesting to note that serotonin is implicated in this disorder. By consuming food that can be converted to serotonin, we may be able to help ourselves resist the temptations of normal food cravings; at least, that is what my patients tell me.

Your snack should be a food that will benefit your body and that you find satisfying. By the latter, I mean there are times when you might want a food with a creamy consistency—in such a case, low-fat yogurt is a great choice. At other times, you may desire a crunchy texture—here I would suggest baby carrots or raw celery stalks. And don't forget to drink at least one 8-ounce glass of water; this assures that you are not misinterpreting the signal for thirst as a hunger signal.

Purchase a stopwatch and try these techniques. They will lead you to the realization that you are powerful and that your willpower is stronger than you now believe. After a month or so you may not need the stopwatch because you will have truly overcome the lure of cravings. You will find that the power was within you all along and you just needed to stop and watch for it to appear.

Stop! Watch! Method Summary

1. Set your watch or a timer for 15 minutes.
2. Drink a large glass of water
3. Eat a high-protein snack.

HIGH-CALCIUM POWER SNACKS STOP CRAVINGS

Tryptophan is a natural craving stopper!

At Nighttime

Make sure that your snack is calcium rich! Dairy products are your best bet because they are high in L-tryptophan and calcium. Calcium has been shown to benefit weight reduction and it is also a natural sleeping aid. Try a glass of skim milk (perhaps with a sprinkling of cinnamon, which helps control insulin), some fat-free yogurt, or low-fat cheese prior to retiring. These snacks stop cravings, strengthen your bones, and help you to lose weight, while you sleep.

During the Day

Avoid simple carbohydrates: no cookies or cake with your milk! These will raise blood sugar and stimulate hunger. Avoid chocolate: It, too, raises blood sugar and contains caffeine. Anyone who is a parent and has been forced to deal with a child who has had too much Halloween candy can attest to the stimulant effect of sweets! You want protein, which is ultimately far more satiating.

POWER SNACKS

- Organic peanut butter (1 tablespoon) spread on apple slices combines all three food groups: protein and healthy fat from the peanut butter, and complex carbohydrates with fiber from the apple.

(continued)

- ½ cup of low-fat or skim ricotta cheese with ¼ cup of berries provides protein, calcium, complex carbohydrates with fiber, and a small amount of fat.
- Almonds and walnuts are delicious, high in the good kind of fat, and will curb your appetite. You must exercise self-control, however, as they are also high in calories. I suggest dividing a can of nuts into sealed portion-size bags. If you work in an office, keep these in your desk—they will prevent you from raiding the candy jar. If you are at home during most of the day, this trick will save you from eating more than you should.
- A 4-ounce can of wild Alaskan salmon or tuna mixed with wasabi mustard and freshly cut-up vegetables used as dip. The small tuna cans with easy-to-open pop-tops are the perfect snack size.
- Hard-boiled omega-3 egg with mustard
- 2 ounces of low-fat cheese with 1 cup raw vegetables

BEGIN YOUR DAY WITH PROTEIN

A study of overweight adolescent boys found that when they started the day with a breakfast of eggs, they reported less hunger before lunch and consumed fewer calories than did a comparison group of boys who had cereal for breakfast. Make your breakfast high protein and you will cut your desire for snacks!

THE NIGHT EATING NURSE

Deborah is a forty-eight-year-old nurse and married mother of two. When she first visited me, she was depressed and frustrated about her inability to lose weight. Deborah had worked for several years as a nursing supervisor on the night shift. During her hospital years, she had struggled by on too little sleep and kept herself alert by eating carbohydrates. After her children were born, she switched to the day shift. Although relieved to be on the same time clock as everyone else, she found it difficult to stay asleep at night and therefore would get up to watch television. While watching television, she would eat.

As time went by Deborah had gained more than 25 pounds. She dieted and lost some weight only to regain it. She could not seem to lose more than 5 to 7 pounds before the scale would not budge. She cut back on her breakfast and usually only had a large cup of coffee in the morning. But even though she was good as gold during the day and ate a reasonable dinner, her habitual night eating caused her to retain weight.

Deborah exhibited three patterns of cravings:

1. She ate when her energy was low. When she was a nursing supervisor, she had set up the pattern of carbohydrate snacking during energy slumps.
2. After her night job had ended, she ate while she was bored during the evening. Her snacks were sweet and highly processed foods.
3. She had created within herself the night eating syndrome.

There was only one answer for Deborah: to stop eating at night. She initially resisted, as she had come to enjoy those late-night old movies! I pointed out that they were easily obtainable on DVDs that she could watch at any hour, and that

(continued)

her snacking on cookies while she watched was the reason for her weight plateau! Deborah agreed to eat a good breakfast and committed to an early-morning workout. The morning workouts were important, because it is virtually impossible to stay up late if you have a 6:00 A.M. workout with a trainer! Deborah threw out the cookies and substituted protein snacks to tide her through the rough times. After a challenging three-week period, her cravings were gone and Deborah had beaten the night eating syndrome. She kept herself satisfied with frequent meals. She is now a sleek 25 pounds lighter. Deborah is happier, healthier, and in control.

Like Deborah, if you are stuck in the vicious cycle of weight gain-loss-gain, make a conscious effort to break the cycle. These situations do not improve by themselves. You need to take control of your environment. For starters, throw out anything that is a processed food and have only the best fresh food available. If you are at home during the day, this means no cookies or crackers. If you are in an office, make sure that your desk is carb free! Have healthy power snacks ready for when the hunger hits. Apply the Stop! Watch! Method to change your snacking pattern.

It is all about planning and thinking ahead, as you already do in other areas of your life. Just apply the same concepts to food. I absolutely guarantee that this will work. It will not work overnight; usually nothing worth having happens overnight. Day by day, week by week, each time you make a choice for a healthy snack you will reinforce within yourself that new behavior. You may slip, but be assured that it is only that, a slip and not a failure.

DIANNE'S TABLE STRATEGIES

The importance of planning ahead is best illustrated by Dianne, a successful and dynamic mover and shaker in the world of public relations. When Dianne first visited me she was overweight and very unhappy. She had tried many diets but to no avail. She was tired all the time, her skin was dry, and the weight that she had gained was distributed around her middle. For a woman accustomed to being in the limelight, this was a most unhappy state of affairs.

Dianne accepted my suggestion of a high-protein and high-calcium diet, and agreed to begin every morning with an aerobic workout. Because she ate virtually every dinner out, her assistant became adept at calling restaurants in advance to order a platter of crudités for the table instead of a bread basket.

The changes that took place with Dianne were truly remarkable. After one month, she had lost 12 pounds. The fact that she saw results gave her incentive to continue and make even greater changes. She installed a small office refrigerator, where she stored her bottles of water and her snack of yogurt with sliced vegetables. After two months, Dianne had lost 20 pounds, but, more important, she intuitively understood that restructuring her environment was what had taken them off. It is difficult to maintain a weight loss if you are surrounded by bad food. Dianne created an environment that worked for her health.

Because entertaining clients was such an important part of Dianne's work, she also came up with a restaurant seating plan that worked to her advantage:

Rao's restaurant, in New York, is noted for its great food and impossible-to-obtain reservations. Dianne was a regular at Rao's, an exclusive restaurant where it is virtually impossible to obtain a table even for celebrities. The restaurant is small and a who's who of the New York scene. On any given night it is not unusual to see Mayor Bloomberg, Broadway stars, Yankees, or even former president Bill Clinton. The seating in the restaurant is in

(continued)

U-shaped booths and the delicious Italian food is served family-style. Dianne quickly realized that if she took an inside seat in the booth, it was far more difficult to eat only her own simple salad topped with grilled shrimp and pass up the homemade pasta that Rao's is famous for. So she made a point of arranging her guests so that she was seated on the outside of the booth. The pasta passed right by her untouched!

I have many patients who have adopted Dianne's seating strategy. It is common sense not to let yourself be surrounded by people pushing you to taste their entrées when you are trying to lose weight. Dianne took control of her environment, rather than letting her environment control her.

Eating out is *de rigueur* among my patients. To empower them, I often suggest that they check out the restaurant ahead of time. The Web site www.menupages.com has menus from restaurants all over Manhattan. My patients can tell me where they will be eating, and I use this site to give them guidelines in advance. They also use this site themselves as a source to choose a restaurant that is more likely to serve healthy choices, so they can stick with their plan. For example, Aureole 34 is a favorite destination for many of my upscale patients, for business entertaining and special events. It is a beautifully romantic hot spot on East Sixty-first Street. One of Aureole's unique features is their Simple Grills over Oak Charcoal menu that offers portobello mushrooms, salmon, tuna, steak, pork, and chicken breast served with simple herb-grilled vegetables and a potato tart. I suggest that my clients ask for steamed vegetables and skip the potato side dish. To start, I will often choose the Salad of Seasonal Lettuces and Herbs with balsamic vinegar as a dressing on the side. Mission accomplished!

WHEN EATING OUT

CUISINE	TIPS
French	Watch out for butter, sauces, carbs, and hidden fats. On the positive side, the portions tend to be manageable. Strategy: Don't eat the bread, and always leave food on your plate.
Italian	As long as you avoid pasta, you are home free! Begin your meal with a fresh salad and balsamic dressing— baby spinach with shaved Parmesan cheese and balsamic vinegar is delicious at Brio in New York City. There is nothing better than fish prepared Mediterranean style. End the meal with espresso or skim cappuccino.
Chinese	Choose steamed over stir-fried or sautéed vegetables, chicken, shrimp; avoid anything fried, and stick with brown rice only if you are at the phase 2 level; if you are at phase 1, don't eat any rice at all.
Japanese	Miso soup, seaweed salad, and tofu salad are nutritious first courses. As far as fish goes, sashimi is better than sushi. However, if you ask for your sushi to be made with a small amount of rice, most spots will happily oblige. Hibachi-grilled fish, chicken, or beef is a good choice as well. Avoid tempura and noodles. Order green tea.
Thai	Avoid anything with coconut milk, which is very high in saturated fat. Pad Thai is one of the most fattening dishes you can eat.
Mexican	Stick with fish, salsa, black beans, or guacamole with vegetables. As long as you avoid food that is fried and covered with cheese, you'll be safe.
Cuban	The fish soups are magnificent. Meats and chicken are usually marinated in garlic and herbs, often on the spicy side. Choose the delicious marinated and grilled main

(continued)

CUISINE	TIPS
	courses; they have the Cuban essence and will save you calories. Avoid empanadas and doughy choices.
Mediter-ranean	Olive oil, olive, and tomato–based tapenades are delicious starters. The Mediterranean diet is one of the healthiest diets in the world. Watch portion sizes.
Vegetarian	Be careful; vegetarian menus are loaded with grains and carbs.
Steakhouse	Everyone visits a steakhouse sometime. You know what to expect: a big bread basket, too much meat, a large potato with butter, and a vegetable with too much butter. Here you risk a coronary if you don't speak up and order what will be the best choice. Ask for filet mignon, cut it in half, and request that your vegetable be butter free. Eat neither bread nor potato. Start with a salad and have the dressing on the side.

Avoiding Saboteurs

One of the challenges in sticking to this program or any other, is dealing with the well-meaning "saboteurs" who are at the ready to steer you off course. For example, the boyfriend who doesn't want to drink alone. Or the girlfriend who complains that you are "getting too thin," or the well-meaning relative who says you are "just skin and bones." DON'T LISTEN TO THEM. Stay firm in your commitment to sticking with your program. At the bottom of this is the fact that people just do not like change. They will do anything to maintain the status quo. There is something threatening in seeing someone change: Your friends fear that you will disapprove of their food choices or alcohol consumption when you are thinner; they fear you will find new friends who are more fun. Your lover fears rejection as your body becomes thinner, and is afraid that you may find a superior lover. It may seem irrational, but change magnifies insecurities in all of us. Out of fear, and often without realizing it, your friends may begin to fight the change that has taken place in you. This fear is universal and I witness it almost daily in my practice, so I advise my patients to prepare for it. The truth is: All these fears may prove to be real! You may very well find a whole new group of healthier, slimmer friends or stop eating lunch with the people who overeat; you may even find a more attractive, nicer, and more successful lover. But the chances are that you will keep the relationships that are now present in your life.

Your goal is to remain focused. It is a worthy one: You have the goal of health and to make your body as fit and strong as it can be. Even if your friends and loved ones make it harder to stay on track, you must because there is no other way. This is for *your* life and for *your* health.

Lucy is one of the most vital and exciting people that I have ever known. She is a forty-one-year-old magazine editor who has traveled the world, can talk with anyone about any subject, and has even dated a crown prince. I met her at a dinner party and, while she is slim, her husband whom she adores is quite heavy. When Lucy discovered that my medical practice is devoted to nutrition and weight reduction, she insisted that her husband see me. Her husband, Roger, age sixty-three, dutifully complied. As he followed the program, he gradually began to lose weight. It was not easy for him—as he was the head of a major advertising firm, his frequent entertaining was a large part of his and Lucy's lifestyle. But he incorporated the principles that I have described into his life and, miracle of miracles, he even joined a gym.

Roger became a new man! His sex life with Lucy improved. He bought new clothes. He became healthy; his cholesterol declined by 50 points as he lost 40 pounds. In every way, the changes that occurred within Roger were wonderful and, indirectly, benefited Lucy. Her husband was sexier, and was going to probably live longer than if he had continued on his previous

(continued)

course. Everywhere they went, people complimented Roger. Now he was in the limelight. So quite unknowingly, Lucy became a saboteur. She ordered his favorite desserts (a great temptation for Roger) and suggested that he take just a taste; she left cookies around the apartment and encouraged Roger to stay out late, giving him a reason to miss his new 6:00 A.M. workout. Lucy did not intentionally want to make her husband fall off his plan but, because of all the attention the new and improved Roger got, she no longer felt like the star.

When Roger and I talked about the problem, I made the suggestion that he just sit down with Lucy and let her know how her behavior was hurting him. He needed to reassure her that she was the love of his life. He told her that, after a while, people would get used to seeing his new body; it would not always be a novelty and that she would always shine brightly. It was important that Roger bring the issue out into the open and acknowledge that he had threatened Lucy's position as the main attraction at a party. If this had continued, marital problems could have resulted and Roger could have regained his weight and lost his wife and his health.

Chapter Six

THE STOP! WATCH! METHOD

OF EXERCISE

*To be "fit as a fiddle," you must tone up
your middle.*

• • •

Daily physical activity is a basic element of good health. Indeed it should be a way of celebrating life and the ability to move. If you are fortunate enough to have the gift of being able to use your limbs (and many people cannot), then it is incumbent upon you not to to fall into disrepair. Your body requires exercise to maintain its optimal performance level. Without physical exercise, you will look and feel older than your chronological age. This is a well-documented scientific fact.

What this comes down to is preserving and enhancing your greatest asset: yourself. You deserve to—and must—give yourself the best care. To accomplish this, you must make exercise part of every day, at a regular, specific time, preferably prior to breakfast. People who work out in the morning are 40 percent more likely to maintain this than those who postpone their workout until later in the day.

Whatever fitness level you are now at, you can improve. As with your food intake, having a plan can help you succeed. If you have not done any sort of exercise since riding your bicycle to school, begin slowly. But you must begin—and you must do it consistently. You will delight in your new strength and endurance as you make this a daily part of your life.

The single best thing an individual over forty years of age can do for his or her health is to commit to daily exercise. You can actually halt the aging process by doing so. Sweat is the elixir of youth! I mean this very seriously.

> *If you are fifty or more years of age and have not exercised at all, consult with your physician before beginning an exercise program.*

Weeks 1 to 4

Begin your day with an aerobic workout. It does not matter what activity you choose, whether it is running outdoors or jogging on the treadmill or using a real or stationary bicycle or going for a brisk walk. What matters is consistency, that you find an activity that you enjoy and stay with it. This means even on those mornings when you don't want to get out of bed, you still get up and exercise. It won't work if you just do it when you feel like it. In time, you'll like it. This is often the best part of my day. Once you commit to this, you have given yourself a health advantage and your risks for numerous diseases will fall dramatically.

Just do it, as the Nike slogan says.

Ted, a friend for thirty years, is a fifty-five-year-old dentist. Ted lives in a small Connecticut town where we spend our weekends. He has always exercised and eaten in a health-conscious manner. What is extraordinary about Ted is he gets his exercise in a rather unusual manner. He doesn't bike, ski, jog, or play golf or tennis. Ted goes for strenuous hikes in the beautiful scenery surrounding his home, and lifts weights in his basement. But what sets him apart is that, in his spare time, Ted builds drystone walls!

In case you don't know, drystone walls are constructed by carefully positioning stones together without the use of cement.

(continued)

Stone must be chipped until it fits next to the adjacent stone. The base of the wall is wider than the top, so that the wall will not crumble. Walls constructed in this manner last forever and are very beautiful. Building a stone wall requires strength. The stones used weigh between 50 and 500 pounds. To locate a stone of the correct size and shape is a challenge. After finding appropriate stones in the forest, Ted carries or rolls the stones to his pickup truck, then loads and unloads the stones and positions them artfully as he builds his walls. Ted has become very strong through this weekend exercise. His arms, back, and legs are muscular. He does not have a "spare tire." In fact, our mutual male friends who "exercise" on the golf course look about ten years older than Ted.

Ted has been building stone walls for pleasure since I have known him. He has constructed stone terraces and walks, as well. The graceful walls encircle his lovely estate and have kept him slim and trim through the years.

Find an exercise that you love and just watch where it will take you.

Daily aerobic exercise is the cornerstone of optimum health.

The intensity at which you exercise is important. The standard formula for calculating the maximal heart rate is: 220 minus your age, multiplied by 0.7. However, of late there has been criticism of this formula as underestimating how strenuously an individual may exercise. So I offer to you the following: If you are in good health and are able to carry on a conversation albeit with some heavy breathing, then you are working in the correct aerobic zone. Alternatively, using a scale of 1 to 10, with 10 being the greatest exertion you are capable of, try to keep your level in the range of a 7.

Whatever form of exercise you choose, maintain the idea of challenging yourself. Keep your breathing on the heavy side. You want to work up a sweat.

The duration of activity should be around 45 minutes to an hour, in order to lose weight. But if you don't have this much time to spare, whatever you can do is better than doing nothing at all. Establish the pattern that no matter what happens, you are going to exercise. This is vital. You are creating a new habit. I recommend that you do aerobic exercise on six days out of the week and take one day off for resting.

It is amusing to me to hear my patients say that they don't have the time to exercise for 45 minutes for six days per week. Let me put this in terms my fast-paced patients understand all too well:

- Those 270 minutes represent a small fraction of the week's total of 10,080 minutes; in fact, they are only .026 of a week's time.
- The President of the United States finds time to exercise, and somehow I think that his schedule might be pretty full.
- The health benefits of daily exercise are enormous and the time spent exercising can actually extend your life. So you get a good rate of return back on the investment you make, in terms of your precious time.
- You will look older if you do not exercise and younger if you do.

Set a Goal for Yourself

Week 1. After getting the green light, start with a daily walk of 30 minutes for 1 week. Do this every day for 1 week whether you want to or not. Make consistency your goal for the first week. Your goal is to walk every day for 1 week. Period.

Week 2. During the second week, try alternating jogging and walking—this is where a stopwatch comes in handy. Your new goal is to jog for 1 minute. Begin by walking for 5 minutes just to warm up your muscles, then set the stopwatch for 1 minute and jog for that minute. This does not have to be a run; a slow jog is just fine. It is only a minute, but it may seem like a long time when you first attempt this. Keep jogging until that minute is over and the stopwatch beeps. You will have proven to yourself that you can indeed jog for 1 minute. You have achieved a new goal. Now walk for 5 minutes and repeat the stopwatch sequence again. It won't be easy for you, but you need to challenge your body in order to improve your fitness. If you keep doing the same old thing over and over, you will not be using the time that you have set aside for fitness to its greatest benefit. We all want the most for our money, so let's get the most for our time!

Week 3. I suggest that, after your 5-minute warmup, you set the stopwatch for 90-second jog and 5-minute walk intervals. Week by week, you will use the stopwatch to increase the number of minutes that you jog by 30-second increments. This will allow your body time to adjust to the new physical activity that you are providing to yourself.

Week 4. By now you should set the stopwatch for 2-minute jog and 5-minute walk intervals and increase the total time of your workout to 35 minutes.

Weeks 5 and 6. Increasing your jogging intervals to 30-second intervals, progress to 40 minutes total workout time by the fifth week and 45 minutes by the sixth. Continue to use the stopwatch beyond the 6-week mark. The stopwatch helps you to stay focused, causing you to continue your jog just for those few extra seconds, and keeps track of overall time so you are aware of how long your workout lasts.

In 6 weeks you will be doing more for your body than 85 percent of the American population do for theirs. This is a wonderful change that will have long-reaching benefits for your health, lowering your risks for diabetes, cardiovascular disease, and numerous cancers. What may have started as a difficult and taxing task will have become a powerful source of physical renewal and strength. You will have exchanged the unhealthy habit of inactivity for the health-promoting habit of daily aerobic exercise.

> *By breaking down the task into several manageable goals, you are setting yourself up to succeed. If you had started with a goal of running 45 minutes daily, you would have failed. A realistic goal almost guarantees success.*

I assure you that you will notice a positive change in how you look and feel. You will sleep more soundly, and stress will have less effect on you. If there is a magic bullet, then it surely must be aerobic exercise!

What I have described above is a program for an inactive person to become more fit through a walk/jog interval program. I think this program is applicable to the majority of people, but there are some for whom it is not. If arthritis, spinal stenosis, extreme obesity, or other conditions prevent you from walking for an extended period of time, the program can be adapted to an exercise bicycle in place of the jogging part. The concept remains the same. Just begin the activity and perform it daily at the same time for one week for 30 minutes. To add intervals while biking/walking, just extend the bicycling time. Follow the same progression that is described for jog/walk until you are working out for 45 minutes at the end of 6 weeks.

If you need extra motivation, enlist a friend to walk or jog with you, or hire a personal trainer. Whatever it takes, get yourself going! You are less likely to cancel if you have an appointment with someone.

Working with a Trainer

In addition to daily aerobic exercise on your own, hire a trainer. The benefit of working out with a personal trainer is plain and simple: He or she will push you harder than you will push yourself. On those mornings when you stayed out too late the night before and would skip working out in favor of sleeping in, the trainer will force you to exercise. If you can afford it, you should give yourself this extra motivator. Trainers are expensive, but they are worth every penny if you are out of shape and haven't exercised in a while. When exercising with weights and machines, it is crucial that your alignment be correct, or injury could result. An experienced personal trainer will look for this and correct your form as necessary.

I recommend that you work only with a trainer who is certified by the American College of Sports Medicine, the National Academy of Sports Medicine, or the National Strength and Conditioning Association. Experienced trainers will have multiple certifications. The personal trainer that you work with should be someone with whom you have a rapport and trust. It is not helpful to you if they are overly chatty or seek your professional advice during training sessions.

Optimally, you should work out with your personal trainer three times per week. If you want to work out on your own, then consult a trainer to put together a program for you, and see the trainer every month for updates to your program as you get stronger.

Endorphins Are Addictive!

The bottom line is it really doesn't matter what you do so much as the intensity of effort and consistency of training are what increase fitness. Just pick an activity and do it. You may not even enjoy it that much in the beginning; my patients frequently ask, "How long does it take before I start to like this?" The answer to that question is different for everyone. As anyone who has made a commitment to daily exercise will tell you, it is very addictive; once you have begun, you will both look forward to your workout and miss it when it is an impossibility to do it. Why? During exercise, your body produces chemicals called endorphins. Endorphins are similar to a class of pain-relieving drugs called opiates. Endorphins interact with the opiate receptors in the brain and cause feelings of euphoria. Prolonged, continuous release of endorphins is responsible for "runner's high." When you work out regularly you may find that the natural high you experience gives you a lift and helps you cope with everyday problems more productively. So, besides the considerable physical benefits, there are also tremendous psychological benefits of exercise!

Exercise Yourself Young

A recent 2-year study followed fifty early-postmenopausal women who exercised intensely—they performed two group exercise and two home exercise sessions per week. These women were compared to a group of women of similar age and health who did not exercise. At the conclusion of the 2 years, significant beneficial effects of exercise were found: Physical fitness as isometric strength had increased by 35 percent, oxygen consumption by 12 percent, bone density in both the spine and hip has increased significantly, and cholesterol had gone down. The women who did not exercise had the opposite result in the 2-year period: their strength declined, oxygen consumption and bone density worsened, and their cholesterol went up.[1]

By consistently exercising, the women in the first group had side-stepped the aging process. Their bones, muscles, and hearts were comparable to those of women who were younger. The women who did not exercise had a decline in their bodies reflecting a greater age than they were chronologically. By not exercising, they had prematurely aged!

Sex and Exercise

If the benefits that I have already mentioned aren't enough to get you into the exercise groove, perhaps knowing that regular physical exercise will improve your sex life will motivate you. Because exercise improves circulation to all body parts, including the genitals and pelvic region, it seems logical that exercise would affect sexual activity. Exercise also increases the amount of blood that we produce, which seems conducive to erectile functioning.

In the Massachusetts Male Aging Study, which followed men age forty to seventy over several years, those who were regular exercisers had sex more frequently than men who didn't exercise. A study from the University of California, San Diego, looked at the quality of sex associated with exercise: When sedentary middle-aged men started exercising three to four times per week, for an hour at a time, they reported firmer erections, better orgasms, and greater frequency of sexual intercourse. The Health Professionals Study followed more than 31,000 males between the ages of fifty-three and ninety, and assessed through the use of questionnaires the frequency of their sexual activity and their amount of physical exercise.[2] Men over age fifty who remained physically active had a 30 percent lower risk of impotence than did men who were inactive.

> *The fitter the man, the better the erection.*

The results for women are not as well documented but a University of Texas study of women age eighteen to thirty-four found that after an exercise session blood flow to the vagina increased over 150 percent, thus enhancing sexual response after workouts.

The positive benefits of exercise for males and females give an important message: Sexual activity can stay strong and provide years of enjoyment through committing to daily aerobic exercise. Loss of sexuality is not part of normal aging, but rather a response to a sedentary lifestyle.

> *The message is get moving and stay young!*

Additional Exercise Programs

The Central Park Walking Program

I have devised a route for my Manhattan patients to follow that allows them to experience the natural beauty of Central Park while exercising. (You can find this in chapter 2.) Studies have shown that being in a natural surrounding can actually lower your heart rate, decrease tension, and improve focus and concentration. The beauty of nature is a balm for the soul. Wherever you live, city or country, you can find a setting that rejuvenates your spirit. The flat plains of the Texas Panhandle, the steep hills of San Francisco, the early-morning desert of Las Vegas, the snowy plains of Minnesota in winter: All are majestic natural gymnasiums. Just grab your sneakers, bicycle, cross-country skis, or snowshoes and off you go to a healthier, stronger, and younger new body!

The Half-Hour Strengthening Program

Besides aerobic activity, we need activity that challenges our muscles and makes us stronger. Women often are afraid that they will become too muscular and look like weight lifters. This is just simply not the case. Women who are bodybuilders work out with heavy weights for hours daily. What will occur is that your arms will lose the "bridge party" flap of skin, your thighs won't jiggle, and your hips and waist will become firmer. You will become stronger and sleeker. You will probably go down in dress size; your clothes will drape more gracefully.

Begin with a 2- to 3-minute warmup. Stand tall and lift one knee and then the other to your chest while swinging the opposite arm forward, thirty times. This elevates your heart rate, increases the circulation to the large muscles of the legs, and engages the abdominal muscles. Warm up the back and abdominal muscles with rotation movements: Hold your abdominal muscles in tightly and with your feet at shoulder-distance apart, reach your arms down to your right side, then with arms extended reach over your left shoulder. Do this ten times on each side of the body. Now you are ready to begin your half-hour strength program. Always warm up before beginning!

Upper Body

Either weights or resistance bands may be used. Better yet, use weights for one session and at the next session use bands. By alternating the form of resistance, you give yourself a little extra challenge.

Bicep curls. Use 5-pound weights and do twelve repetitions. Do a lower-extremity exercise and then repeat.

Or if you prefer, you can use light (usually green) resistance bands; these give a comparable amount of resistance to the weights. Stand on the tubing with your feet directly under your hips and, with palms facing upward, do twelve bicep curls. Keep your shoulders back and down. Your elbows should be pressing into your waist. Repeat after a lower-extremity exercise.

Overhead shoulder reaches. Use 2-pound weights and do twelve repetitions. Keep your shoulders back and down as you raise your arms. Do a lower-extremity exercise, then repeat.

Tricep extensions. Using one of the 5-pound weights, grasp it with both hands and, raising it overhead, hold it behind your back. Keep your elbows at your ears, back straight, abdominals tight, and raise the weight over your head with both hands. Lower behind your back. Do twelve repetitions.

Alternate these three exercises for a total of two sets on each side.

If you prefer, you can use the green bands. Stand on the tubing, with one foot in front of the other foot. Bend at the waist; keeping your back straight and your elbow at your side, extend your arm. Do twelve repetitions on each arm. Repeat.

That's it for the upper body.

Lower Body

Squats. With your feet hip-width apart, bend your knees and reach your bottom backward until you are in a squatting position. Your knees should be over your toes, or you risk stressing your knees. Keep your back straight. Do twelve repetitions. Alternate with an upper-extremity exercise.

Side-lying leg raises. Lie on your right side and bend your right knee; raise your left leg as high as possible and then lower it. Keep your body straight and do not allow your hip to roll inward. Hip and shoulders should be in a straight line. Do twelve repetitions on each side.

Alternate these two exercises for a total of two sets.

That's it for the lower body.

Chest

Chest press. Lying on your back, with your arms bent at 90 degrees and extended out to the side, bring the 8-pound weight over your chest with your arms fully extended. Slowly lower to the starting position. Do fifteen repetitions.

Chest flies. With your arms at your sides while holding the 5-pound weights in each hand, bring them across your chest, as though you are hugging a big ball, and then slowly lower out to the sides again. Do fifteen repetitions.

To use bands to do chest flies, use the loop to attach the band to a closed door, then step away until you feel a challenging resistance on the band. With arms bent and extended at the side, bring them forward as though you are holding a big ball. Do fifteen repetitions. Repeat.

Repeat both exercises.

Torso

> **Crunches**. With knees bent and your fingers crossed behind your head, raise your shoulders off the floor. Do not bend your neck forward but rather keep your eyes focused on the ceiling. Slowly lower down. Do thirty repetitions.

> **Cross-overs**. Lying on the floor with knees bent, cross one ankle over the opposite knee and, with your fingers crossed behind your head, raise the opposite shoulder to the knee. Keep the other shoulder on the floor. Do twenty repetitions on each side.

Back

Lying on your stomach and looking down at the floor, extend your arms in front of you and raise the right arm off the ground while also raising the left leg. Perform the movement with the left arm and right leg. Alternate the right and left side until you have done a total of ten extensions. Rest for 15 seconds and repeat for another ten extensions.

Balance

Balance training should be part of your workout. Stand on one leg for 30 seconds, then balance on the opposite leg for 30 seconds. When this gets too easy, try doing it with your eyes closed!

A Stability Ball

That is all there is to it. You have strengthened your entire body. Once you have mastered these moves, I suggest that you incorporate a stability ball. The stability ball is a top piece of equipment because it causes you to tighten your abdominal muscles during each sequence. The stability ball forces you to work on balance. Once you have mastered the exercises, do your bicep curls, tricep extensions, and overhead shoulder reaches while seated on the ball. Sitting on the ball will narrow your base of support. Once you have mastered this, try lifting one foot off the floor. This will narrow your base of support even more. The ball may be used for abdominal curls and back extensions as well. Using a stability ball does not add extra time to your workout.

Extra Weights

When the 5-pound weights don't challenge you enough, move up to 8-pound weights for biceps and triceps for some of the repetitions. Do this gradually and soon you will find that you will be able to perform your entire workout with the heavier weights. Caution: Do not increase the weights of the overhead shoulder reaches, as the shoulders are smaller muscles and cannot lift as heavy a load as the biceps or triceps.

Jump Rope

When you have mastered the above exercises, add the jump rope. You should not jump rope if you have osteoporosis or ankle, knee, or hip problems. But if these conditions are not present, you should know that jumping rope is the single best all-around exercise one can do. It builds bone, is a great cardio workout, and helps with coordination. Start with just 30 seconds and work up to 5 minutes. (Remember when you were a kid and you spent hours jumping rope?)

> *And that is all there is to this very simple method of strengthening your entire body!*

TOP FAT BURNERS

- Jumping rope
- Treadmill
- Nordic Track
- Rowing Machine

Join a gym. Personally, I love the energy of working out with others. The weather is never a consideration and cannot be used as an excuse for not working out. Gyms have all sorts of new and unusual classes: spinning, dancing, aerobic interval classes, and so on. The Equinox Fitness Clubs have one called Brazilian Butt Lift that is sensationally popular! Just try them all until you find one that suits you best. I like to take different classes that are new to me; it keeps things interesting. Use the machines, with your trainer's guidance.

The Park Avenue Plan to Get Moving

Both the Central Park walking program and the strengthening program were designed to introduce my Park Avenue patients to a more active lifestyle. These programs involve aerobic and resistance activity. But there are certain mind-sets that determine how we respond to exercise. By this I mean that we are each unique, complex individuals with our own preferences. Psychologically, we need to tailor our workouts to our personalities. It is possible to use the physical challenge of your workout to change your emotional state. This is more than just the endorphin boost that follows physical exertion. The exercise that you choose to do can change the limitations that you see for yourself. If you try an activity that requires you to think in a different way, you will develop new physical and mental strength.

Running

For individuals who have difficulty completing projects or a fear of commitment, running is a sport to consider. You are required to focus for the time that you are doing it. As you stay with it, you get better. The act of running is a challenge that leaves you gasping for breath initially. But if you stick with it, distances that once appeared endless are easily finished. Your body overcomes the urge to stop as your mind tells you to keep going. The NYC Marathon is filled with people whose bodies say, "Stop!" but whose minds say, "Keep going!"

If commitment is your weak point, give running a try. You can build your ability to commit. Running positively reinforces the concept of hard work paying off by allowing you to go farther and farther with each run.

Running is great for showing yourself your own ability to persist and to complete the run. At first, it seems a miracle to finish 2 miles, then 5 miles. You know that if you try you could run for 10 miles. And so you do.

Victor, who was having difficulty staying with his diet plan, decided to enter a 4-mile race. He had been accustomed to running 3 miles several times a week and he was advised by colleagues that it was perfectly all right to walk for the difficult portions of the course. But Victor thought to himself, "If I really have trouble, there is no way that I am going to just walk! I will just run off to the side and exit the race. I don't have to complete the course." As Victor was going up the most difficult hill of the race, he observed several runners walking up the hill. Later, these runners resumed running and several easily passed Victor.

Victor thought about this, and reasoned one does not always have to run. The point is to complete the race. He completed the race and applied the concept to his diet plan. He stayed with it. Even though his weight loss had slowed, he persisted. He eventually reached his weight loss goal.

Kickboxing

For individuals who lack confidence and feel that they are easily pushed around, kickboxing is a good sport. Kickboxing releases pent-up aggression through power strikes. More and more females are taking up kickboxing. Several years back, kickboxing was exclusively a male sport. But both males and females can benefit from the aggressive release obtained in its quick, powerful movements.

As children, girls were often told to "behave" and not exhibit aggressive behavior. Later in life, women may discover that they don't have the skills needed to take a stance. Deep within their subconscious is heard the voice of a parent telling them, "Behave like a lady" or "Don't be a tomboy." In the past, female role models were often passive. But in the workplace, passivity is not the most desirable quality. One needs to have "fire in the belly" to succeed. By taking up a sport that forces one to become aggressive, one is able to "practice" the ability to assert oneself.

Yoga

If you tend to be impulsive, competitive, and overly aggressive, yoga is a solution worth trying. The moves of yoga are controlled, strong, and relaxing. Yoga causes you to focus inward, concentrate on your breathing, and let go of stress. If your tendency is to be on overdrive, yoga allows you to relax and meditate. The discipline of yoga is directly inward; you focus on and balance your emotional and physical strength. You become aware of your breath and are in the moment. You let go of stress.

The poses may be done anywhere as a short break in a busy and stressful day.

It Is Natural to Be Active

It is all about the journey, not the destination. It is very unnatural to be inactive. We are designed to run, walk, and live our lives actively. Modern life encourages us to the opposite. Recently, I spoke with a woman who planned an entire wedding without leaving her living room! She did it by telephone and the Internet. Even five years ago this would have been impossible. The point is, our lifestyle of the modern day makes it possible to do everything with a minimum of movement. By giving in to this, you will give up physical strength. You will gain weight. You will look old, flabby, and fat.

Chapter Seven

ANTI-AGING NUTRITION:
LIVE LONGER AND
LOOK YOUNGER

It does change, the age that is young.
Once in Paris it was 26, then it was 22.
Now it is between 30 and 40 that one is
considered young.

—GERTRUDE STEIN

• • •

Fifty is the new thirty, when it comes to age. There is so much more known now than twenty years ago about nutrition and physical activity, it is indeed possible to slow down the aging process or to "turn back time," in the words of that famous over-fifty baby boomer, Cher.

Midlife represents a time of life when some degree of financial security has been achieved and the demands of parenthood have somewhat lessened. I encourage my patients who have reached this stage to use this time to put into place new behaviors that improve their health and extend their lives. While we could get away with poor eating habits and late-night revelry when we were in our twenties, with time these behaviors become more detrimental to our health. How many times have you heard someone say, "I just can't eat as much as when I was younger or I gain weight" or "It is so much harder for me to lose weight now that I am over forty" or "I used to be able to stay up all night drinking and dancing, but now I feel horrible the next day" or "My tolerance for alcohol has gone to hell in a handbasket!" Your body has less tolerance for abuse, so you need to become a guardian for your health.

This diet is also an anti-aging diet. It allows the body to stop aging prematurely. The typical American diet promotes aging through a high amount of sugar, processed food, and unhealthy fats. Within the body these produce a variety of ill effects: Sugar forms complexes that damage the body's proteins, processed foods create a craving for sweet tastes, and the unhealthy fats clog the arteries.

On a cellular level, optimal nutrients are not provided and damage is done. I am recommending youth-promoting foods that fight cellular damage, encourage cell renewal, rebuild cells that have been damaged, and nourish the body from the inside out. By controlling what you eat you will not only become slimmer, you will look younger.

My diet plan is composed of foods that benefit the body, exercise that strengthens the heart and lungs, and stress-reduction techniques. By leaving behind unhealthy behaviors, we can reverse the pre-illness stage, look younger, and enjoy good health. My plan takes advantage of the advances in nutritional science and allows you to choose foods that maximally benefit the body. And they are all delicious.

In this chapter, I will review the theories of aging and what we can do to stay young for as long as possible.

Why We Age

Why do our bodies change? Why do we show signs of aging? It all comes down to what occurs within the cell. Damage at the cellular level is repaired during youth; but with age, cellular damage accumulates. The exact mechanism of aging is, as of now, undefined. Several theories of interest are still under investigation.

The Telomere Theory

DNA, as everyone knows, carries our genetic code: what color our eyes and hair will be, how tall we will be, what diseases we are predisposed to, and so on. DNA is stored within chromosomes inside every cell of our body. Our cells continually renew themselves throughout our lifetime. Each time a cell is renewed, DNA within the cell makes a copy of itself. The end portion of each chromosome, known as the telomere, has been noted to shorten with time. When we are young, the telomeres are quite long but as we age, due to constant replication, they become shorter and shorter. It has been speculated that the shortening of the telomere accounts for aging of the cell.

Additionally, certain parts of our body age more rapidly than others. Thyroid functions decline, cartilage in knees wears out, our vision changes. It has been hypothesized that telomere shortening is tissue specific. Biopsies from various sites in the body seem to confirm this, with telomeres becoming shorter in these body regions first.

As everyone knows, women live longer than men. It is interesting to note that a study of middle-aged men and women found not only that their telomere length became shorter with age, but also that the telomeres were longer in women than in men of the same age.[1] The longer telomere length in women may mean that, for a given chronological age, biological aging in men proceeds faster than in women.

Does Stress Affect the Cell?

We have all observed how chronically stressed people appear haggard and old, and psychological stress is well known to predispose people to premature aging and diseases associated with aging. If stress causes us to age, might not this be seen at the cellular level as shortened telomeres? This startlingly simple hypothesis was tested by doctors Elizabeth Blackburn and Elissa Epel of the University of California, San Francisco.[2] Following a group of mothers caring for a child with a chronic disorder like cerebral palsy or autism, they examined the DNA and telomere length. When the researchers compared the DNA of mothers caring for disabled children, they found a striking trend: After correcting for the effects of age, the longer the women had cared for a sick child, the shorter their telomere length. Chronic stress was actually shortening the telomere! It is obvious that mothers of ill children would feel enormous stress; this study gave concrete evidence of how it might accelerate aging. Additionally, the mothers' *perceived stress*, or how much stress the women said they felt, was directly proportional to the telomere length. The mothers who rated themselves as being able to cope well and who did not see the stress as overwhelming had longer telomeres.

It is amazing to think that stress, which comes from outside of our bodies, can have an effect on the DNA telomere, deep within the nucleus of the cell. The stress the women felt was aging their bodies beyond what would normally be expected. Using a formula to determine body age from telomere length, the telomeres from mothers with high levels of chronic perceived stress showed their bodies to have aged approximately eleven years beyond their biological age! Thus, a thirty-year-old woman with a high level of perceived stress would have a body age of forty-one. It should be pointed out that this study was done with women. However, telomeres in men shorten faster than in women, resulting in older male body age. It seems reasonable to predict that perceived stress in a male might result in a magnified aging process.

In the future, telomere manipulation may become relevant as research on aging continues. It is thought by some that progressive shortening of the chromosome ends accounts for cellular aging.

Learning to manage stress effectively can minimize the aging effect. Just because stress exists in our life does not mean it has to harm us. Stress is a constant in most people's lives, but the effect of stress varies from individual to individual. We determine if stress is going to harm us or not. The key is to learn to manage it, and I will teach you the stress-management techniques you need. Even if you have never learned to do this effectively until now, you are never too old. These are strategies that can be mastered at any age.

Oxidative Damage

Oxygen is vital for us to live. We breathe approximately twenty times per minute, filling our lungs with this vital gas. Our heart then pumps our blood through the lungs, where a protein called hemoglobin grabs its oxygen and carries it to the cells of our bodies. Within the cells, oxygen is used for energy creation. But this vital process creates byproducts of oxygen metabolism, called "reactive oxygen species." Reactive oxygen species may be thought of as waste products of oxygen metabolism. Harmful to cells, reactive oxygen species can damage proteins, lipids, and DNA, and are found in all cells. Body cells are under continuous oxidative stress just by the process of living and have an extensive network of antioxidant defenses for protection.

As we age, the damage from oxidative stress accumulates and our protective mechanisms cannot keep up. The magnitude of the damage is made worse by environmental factors, such as cigarette smoke, air pollution, lack of sleep, and poor diet. Excessive weight causes oxidative damage to the body. Excessive fat is associated with more oxidative damage through an increase in inflammation.

We can reduce the damage by avoiding active and passive cigarette smoke, getting adequate sleep, and eating an optimal diet. Consumption of antioxidant foods, such as red beans, blueberries, and fresh fish, is vital.

Just as there are antioxidant foods that protect and cleanse the body of toxic damage, there are pro-oxidant foods that promote damage. The top pro-oxidant foods are overly processed foods, high-fructose corn syrup, and high-sugar foods. Sadly, most of us consume these as snack foods. Processed foods with high fructose did not even exist until about forty years ago. This sweetener is now widely used, accounting for more than 40 percent of all sweeteners in food. From 1970 to 2000 its use increased by 1,000 percent. Its introduction into the U.S. food chain parallels the rise in obesity. While fructose in fruit is natural and gives sweetness to berries and all fruits, the effect of high-fructose corn syrup in the body is directly impacted upon the liver with an increased production of fat. Beware of "all-natural" processed foods that slip this sweetener into their product.

THE TOP TEN ANTIOXIDANT FOODS

The FDA has published a list of the top ten antioxidant foods. They fight the oxidative wear and tear that occurs throughout our lives. We must avail ourselves of all opportunities to prevent damage; these foods offer a delicious way of doing so. Take the list with you to the grocery store and be sure to consume a wide variety of the foods, as each fights off harm in a different manner.

1. Small red beans
2. Wild blueberries
3. Red kidney beans

(continued)

4. Pinto beans
5. Blueberries (cultivated)
6. Cranberries
7. Artichokes
8. Blackberries
9. Prunes
10. Raspberries

Note that these foods are of various colors. The colors of foods signify different phytochemicals or antioxidants. Each color fights the aging process in a different manner. The more color you add to your diet, the better.

The Glycation Theory

Did you know that too much sugar and simple carbohydrates can cause aging? To function efficiently, the body keeps blood glucose within a very narrow range. If blood glucose falls too low, we slip into a coma; if blood glucose is too high, diabetes is the result. Excess sugar raises the blood cholesterol. Cholesterol not only comes from diet but is synthesized by the liver; too much sugar increases the synthesis of cholesterol. If you think that you are ahead of the cholesterol game by consuming a low-fat diet composed of processed foods, you are sadly mistaken. Low-fat foods often substitute sugar for the missing fat.

The glycation theory of aging concerns the effect of excessive sugar in the body. Too much sugar binds to proteins within our body, forming unhealthy substances called "glycation products." Glycation products damage the organs. In the eye, these harmful complexes form cataracts; in the arteries, the sugar/protein complexes are part of the atherosclerotic process; even the red blood cell's hemoglobin is harmed by glycation; and the collagen of the skin is disrupted by glycation—resulting in wrinkles.

How much glycation is present in the body is determined by how much the blood glucose is elevated and how long the elevation remains. An occasional sugary dessert is not harmful, but daily consumption of a high-sugar diet will result in a massive deposition of glycation products throughout the entire body.

Likewise, consuming highly processed foods that contain high-fructose corn syrup or partially hydrogenated oils also creates glycation products. Processed foods are deceptive because the labels may state that they are "sugar free" or "low fat," thus tricking consumers into thinking that they have made a healthful choice. Actually, the inclusion in foods of high-fructose corn syrup has been linked to the rise in obesity and diabetes.

We can measure the glycation state by looking at the red blood cell in a simple lab test for glycosalated hemoglobin. Because the red blood cell lives for 3 months, the measurement of the sugar-protein complex in the red blood cell reflects just how much sugar the body is overconsuming. A value over 6 indicates danger of diabetes. A value of slightly less than 6 may mean that while diabetes is not present, the consumption of sugar is too high. It is not sufficient to rely only on the measurement of fasting blood glucose, as this reflects a single isolated measurement, not a 3-month period. If you are overweight, I suggest that you have your hemoglobin tested, even if your fasting glucose is normal. Ask for the test; it is not normally done unless an individual is diabetic. By being tested early and by committing to the diet, you will prevent not only diabetes but other sequelae of the aging process.

A high-sugar diet damages your body from the inside; it subtly changes the proteins of your eyes, nerves, arteries, and skin.

Life Expectancy

Now that we have explained some of the mechanisms of why we age, let's focus on how long we can live.

What Is the Maximum Life Span?

It now appears that the maximum achievable life span is approximately 120 years. This number is derived from studies across all species from wild animals, fruit flies, and Galapagos turtles, which have shown that the maximum achievable life span is approximately six times the number of years from birth to maturity. In humans, assuming that maturity occurs around age twenty, this works out to 120 years.

Historically this has been proven to be the case with the longest-lived human, a French woman named Jeanne Calumet who lived to 122 years. This woman had a great zest for life: She had many friends, was quite socially engaging, and rode her bicycle daily well into her nineties. One of the best quotes I think I have heard was from this lively woman. On the occasion of her hundredth birthday, while being interviewed by a reporter, she stated, "I have only one wrinkle and I sit on it!" This charming remark reveals her spirit and vitality. The manner in which she lived is also instructive: She exercised daily and had many friends. I would like to point out that riding a bicycle requires strength, balance, and good eyesight. Plus, she did it over cobblestones!

The Static Balance Test is an indirect measure of how your body is aging. Best of all, it is a test that you can perform yourself! How long can you stand on one foot with your eyes closed without falling over? People under twenty years old can stand for several minutes. Dr. Roy Walford, a pioneer in the anti-aging movement and author of a book on this subject, suggests the test as a biomarker of our functional age.[3] To test yourself: Stand on a hard surface (not a rug) with both feet together, close your eyes, and lift one foot about 6 inches off the ground, bending your knee at a 45-degree angle. How many seconds can you stand before you have to open your eyes? Your score is an average of three trials. If you can balance for 10 seconds, you are functionally fifty years old or less; if you can balance for 25 seconds, then you are thirty years old or less.

George, a 63-year-old decorator, who followed my diet and exercise program and went from 250 pounds to a trim 185 pounds, at six foot two, was initially able to stand for 10 seconds and now can stand for over 2 minutes!

The island of Okinawa, Japan, also offers clues as to how we might be able to live to a healthy, long life because the longest-lived people on earth reside on this island. People here frequently live to be well over one hundred years old. More importantly, they remain physically active during their later years, as the economy is based on farming. Older people continue to work in the fields as long as they are able. Social structure is strong and age is celebrated. When individuals attain one hundred years, they are paraded throughout their village in beautifully decorated chariots; everyone cheers their length of years and the wisdom that it represents. How different from our own culture, where age is viewed as a handicap.

The lives of the people of Okinawa are characterized by high levels of physical activity throughout the life span, and diets that are high in vegetables and fish as a protein source. In fact, the diet and exercise regimen of the long-lived Okinawa people closely resembles mine! Daily exercise, fresh vegetables, and fish are the common elements between the two plans.

The bodily changes that occur in midlife affect our health and appearance. However, it is possible to reclaim our youth through health-promoting habits. We can turn back the clock! I have witnessed this in hundreds of my patients and in myself.

Age-Related Changes

Changes thought to represent normal physical aging include: a reduction in lean muscle mass, reduction in the respiratory capacity, reduction in bone mass, thinning of the skin, and increase in fat mass.

Let's talk about these age-related changes from head to toe:

The Mind

The mind is what defines us. Our minds contain our history, our aspirations, and our intellect. Of everything that we are, unquestionably the mind is the most important aspect for us to preserve. While it was previously believed that the brain was incapable of forming new neurons in adulthood, that notion has been disproved. In fact, the hippocampus— the center of learning and memory—has the ability to sprout new brain cells at any age in response to mental stimulation.[4]

There are dietary methods that can help us preserve mental clarity.

It is important to eat regularly; do not allow yourself to become overly hungry. The brain requires glucose to think; complex carbohydrates in the form of vegetables and fruit will supply this.

Homocysteine is a substance in the blood that increases the risk for Alzheimer's disease and cardiovascular disease; folic acid, vitamin B_6, and vitamin B_{12} lower it. After age fifty, add a supplement of 400 mcg of folic acid, 1.5 mg of vitamin B_6, and 2.4 mcg of vitamin B_{12}. As we get older, our ability to absorb vitamin B_{12} from food declines, so it is a must to add a supplement.

> *The old saying that "fish is brain food" is true!*

Omega-3 fats, found in fish and plants, are anti-inflammatory. It has been suggested that Alzheimer's disease begins with an inflammatory component.[5] Some studies have shown a reduced risk of Alzheimer's disease among users of anti-inflammatory drugs, such as Motrin and Advil. Inflammation is hypothesized to cause blood vessels to become "leaky," allowing inflammatory proteins to escape and damage brain cells. By consuming anti-inflammatory omega-3 foods, it may be possible for us to prevent the damage before it begins. An additional safeguard is consumption of fish oil capsules—three capsules will give you approximately 1,500 mg of omega-3 fat.

Aerobic exercise is a natural antidote for lagging mental function. Studies of aging people have suggested that low levels of physical activity are associated with an increased risk for cognitive decline over time.[6] Likewise, if we remain physically activity, we maintain our mental abilities. A six-year study of healthy older people found that high cardio respiratory fitness protected against cognitive decline.[7] By remaining physically fit, we reduce our risk for chronic diseases, such as cardiovascular disease, diabetes, and high blood pressure—conditions that are associated with poor mental function in older adults. Also, fitness may be directly associated with cerebral blood flow; optimal cerebral blood flow could mean that the brain is receiving the nutrition and oxygen it requires. Aerobic exercise raises endorphins, the "feel good" brain chemicals, and we think more clearly.

DO SOME BRAIN EXERCISES

Crossword puzzles, arithmetic calculations, card games, taking a class, traveling all stimulate our thinking processes. These are mentally active pursuits, requiring effort on our part. Try walking home along a different route. Study a new language or take dancing lessons. For an individual past the age of fifty, becoming proficient with the computer counts the same as learning a foreign language. The trick is not to be passive by just sitting and watching television.

Hair

Human hair goes through stages of growth and shedding—about 85 percent of our hair being in the growth phase at any one time. Various metabolic conditions (thyroid disease, diabetes, deficiency of vitamin B_{12}, and iron deficiency) can cause hair to be shed at a more rapid rate so that the hair may become quite thin. Hormones can cause hair loss, too; just ask any woman who has ever given birth! Male pattern baldness (characterized by loss of hair at the crown and temples) and female pattern hair loss (characterized by thinning in the frontal and central scalp) are due to decreased hormones.

If the underlying metabolic condition is correctly diagnosed and treated, the hair loss usually resolves and the hair may grow back entirely. The vitamins B_2, E, and C can help. The hair is so sensitive to nutrition that it can be said to be a barometer of our nutritional state. A full and shiny head of hair signals health within the body. Hair loss due to hormonal causes can be treated with a combination of Minoxidil and prescription-strength topical vitamin A.

Wrinkles

As we age, our skin's ability to repair itself is diminished. The sun that we worshiped in our youth leaves its autograph in the way of fine lines and age spots. What can be done: Sunscreen is a must at any age, particularly in middle age. The very best choice for a sun block is zinc oxide because it blocks both UVB rays (these cause sunburn) and UVA (which damages the skin structure and is responsible for photoaging). Zinc oxide is now available in a micronized form that completely disappears into the skin. I suggest that you use this daily—summer and winter—because the damage caused by the sun is cumulative. Can diet affect the skin? Absolutely! The skin is composed of paired strands of collagen held together by vitamin C. When the skin is young and healthy, pairs of collagen bundles are lined up like soldiers. The visible wrinkling of the skin occurs because of disorganization in the alignment of the collagen bundles within the skin. The vitamins A and D promote the realignment of collagen bundles and should be consumed daily.

These vitamins are fat soluble and should not be taken in excess; my recommendation is 5,000 IU of vitamin A and 400 mg of vitamin D, orally. Additionally, vitamins A and D can be applied in topical form, are absorbed through the skin, and can dramatically improve fine surface wrinkling. This is different from expensive creams that promise everything and deliver little. The effects of vitamins A and D have real science to back them up. And they are not expensive. Because each collagen pair is held together by vitamin C, it should also be part of a skin health regimen. Vitamin C should be applied to the surface of the skin daily and a stress dose of vitamin C (250 mg in the morning and 250 mg in the evening) consumed in supplemental form when you are exposed to excessive sun. Vitamin E complements the antioxidant effect of vitamin C. I suggest that you include 400 IU of vitamin E in supplemental form.

Dry, dehydrated, slack skin is not the inevitable effect of aging but rather a reflection of eating foods that promote inflammation and damage. The skin and hair are barometers of every process going on within the body. If we consume a diet that is high in sugar, the skin will reflect this. The body does not tolerate high amounts of sugar; this causes the excessive production of insulin and a process called "glycosylation." This means that the skin is damaged by the constant barrage of sugar in the diet. High amounts of dietary saturated fat predispose the skin to inflammation, whereas the omega-3 fats found in fish have an anti-inflammatory effect. The antioxidants found in vegetables and fruits repair skin damage from the environment and act as natural sunscreens.

Omega-3 fish oils are beneficial for the cardiovascular system and, because they are also anti-inflammatory, have a wonderful effect on the skin. This is something that I have noted entirely by accident in my clinical practice, when I have suggested the consumption of these oils for improvement of the cholesterol profile; my patients reported that their skin seemed "younger looking" and "less dry." When chronic inflammation is present within the body, skin shows the effect of this, as does the cardiovascular system. Skin color becomes mottled, surface capillaries rupture, and puffiness around the eyes and cheeks becomes prominent. Omega-3 oils nourish and hydrate the skin from within, causing the skin to appear less red and smoother. By making fish a staple of your diet, you will prevent skin inflammation. If you don't like fish, I recommend 1,500 mg of omega-3 fish oil daily.

The Midsection

While the abdominal storage of excess weight occurs in males throughout their lives, it is after menopause that females develop this distribution. Fat in the abdomen is dangerous. Abdominal fat is associated with diabetes and increased risk for cardiovascular disease.

Aerobic exercise and reduced calories break down this fat preferentially. Abdominal fat responds quickly to diet and exercise, and you can speed the process by adding 1,200 mg of dairy calcium. Aerobic exercise, reducing total calories, and increasing dairy calcium to 1,200 mg ensure that belly fat is shed and a younger silhouette is revealed.

The Muscles

As we age, the percentage of lean muscle is reduced and we gain weight more easily.

A diet that contains optimal protein is essential. Branched chain amino acids (leucine, isoleucine, and valine) are amino acids that are structurally important in building new muscle. Branched chain amino acids are found naturally in meat and dairy products. I have observed that women tend to limit their intake of protein in favor of carbohydrates. I advise my female patients to add protein at every meal and to include protein snacks. Protein is far more satisfying than carbs and helps to maintain lean body mass. A branched chain amino acid supplement is also helpful. With a challenging combination of resistive exercises for the upper and lower body, muscle mass can be preserved and even increased. This benefit has been observed in people in their seventies and eighties. As we become stronger we feel more energetic; we walk with a bounce in our step and climb the stairs more easily.

Feet

It is sad but true that the one place we could actually use extra fat is the bottom of the foot; but believe it or not, this is where we lose fat as we age. The fat pad on the bottom of the foot thins and our natural cushioning mechanism is lost. Wearing high heels makes this worse because bone growth is stimulated in areas of stress. High heels put the weight of the body on the ball of the foot so that bunions develop. This translates into discomfort while walking and can result in people limiting the amount of time spent walking. And if we become less active, weight gain can occur and cardiovascular fitness decreases. Thus, aching feet can lead to a deterioration of the entire body!

There are many interesting ideas for combating fat pad loss, from collagen injections to fat transfers to the bottom of the foot. Often these procedures make matters worse. I prefer to just advise my patients to avail themselves of comfortable shoes with cushioned soles and to walk as much as possible. Mephistos, Tod's, and Flexa's from Fratelli Rosetti offer great-looking, supremely comfortable walking shoes. When you arrive at your destination, you can put on your Jimmy Choos or Manolo Blahniks!

What is most important as we age is that we preserve our health. Do this in a dynamic, consistent manner and you begin to look and feel younger. I personally am convinced that most of the changes we attribute to "getting older" are preventable and reversible. And who wants to look older than they should?

Jack LaLanne, a well-known fitness guru, could well serve as the poster boy for age being nothing more than a number. Now eighty years old, he maintains his boundless energy and enthusiasm. On his sixtieth birthday, he swam from Alcatraz Island to San Francisco handcuffed and shackled on his legs while pulling a 1,000-pound boat. On his seventieth, he towed seventy boats for a mile and a half. And why did he perform these feats? "To show that anything in life is possible. What the mind can conceive the body can do," he said.

Whatever our age, we have the capability to find ways for challenging our bodies and minds. The more we do, the more we grow. The reverse is also true, and I have seen far too many people who just simply give up.

Other Anti-Aging Measures

Anti-aging medicine is a new frontier and offers great promise. It is based on the premise that there are proactive procedures and treatments that can delay or prevent the decline of aging. This makes sense to me. You need to be aware, however, that all medicines have side effects and caution must be exercised. There is no magic pill, or I would be taking it myself!

Growth Hormone
Human aging is characterized by a reduction in lean muscle mass, reduction in bone mass, thinning of the skin, and increase in the percentage of body fat. Aging has an effect on the secretion of human growth hormone, with its amount declining approximately 14 percent per decade after age thirty. Since the effect of growth hormone in the body is the opposite of the aging process, it has been theorized that administration of the hormone might be able to reverse the aging process. A study by D. Rudman et al., published in *The New England Journal of Medicine* in 1990, hinted that this might indeed be the case![8] In the study twelve healthy men, sixty-one to eighty-one years of age, received growth hormone for 6 months. The administration of growth hormone resulted in a 10-pound increase in lean body mass, a 7-pound decrease in fat mass, and an increase in bone density and skin thickness. But the men also had an increase in their blood pressure and fasting glucose—raising their risk for cardiovascular disease and diabetes.

Another study followed eighteen healthy men sixty-five to eighty-two years of age, who underwent progressive strength training for 14 weeks, followed by an additional 10 weeks of strength training plus either the growth hormone or placebo.[9] In that study, resistance exercise training increased muscle strength significantly; the addition of growth hormone did not result in any further improvement.

Naturally, our growth hormone is released in the body in a pulsatile manner, with the peak occurring during sleep. The artificial administration of the growth hormone is by subcutaneous injection twice per week. The side effects include carpal tunnel syndrome, rising blood pressure, and rising glucose. Such treatment is very expensive, costing approximately $20,000 per year.

While the connection between reversing the aging process and administration of growth hormone may prove to be real, currently there just doesn't appear to be justification that merits the associated risks. More studies are needed before this hormone can be recommended on a large scale. Regular aerobic activity may translate to the equivalent benefit of growth hormone administration without the risks involved. Going to the gym is cheaper, gives equivalent benefits, and doesn't involve risk.

Testosterone

Testosterone is the primary male sex hormone. It is responsible for the emergence of the secondary sexual characteristics: Muscles become stronger, facial hair grows, bone mass increases, the voice deepens, and libido increases. Older men have lower blood concentrations of testosterone than do young men. Aging in men is not associated with an abrupt cessation of gonadal hormone (as is the case with females) but rather with a gradual decline. Effects of low testosterone levels include decreases in muscle mass, muscle strength, bone mass, libido, and erectile function, and impaired mood and sense of well-being. Older men have increased body fat, particularly visceral fat. Testosterone replacement therapy decreases fat mass, increases lean body mass, improves strength, and increases bone mineral density. It enhances libido but does not improve erectile dysfunction.

The Institute of Medicine is currently investigating the use of testosterone replacement therapy in aging. The obvious concerns with testosterone replacement are prostate cancer and prostate enlargement.

Caloric Restriction

Caloric excess is associated with a decrease in life span, as shown in population studies. It is also true that populations with lower-calorie diets live longer. The problem with population studies is that they are not able to isolate a single factor as being causative; there may be other environmental factors that are at play. However, in the United States both the Harvard Alumni Health Study[10] and the Nurses Health Study[11] have linked a lower body weight with a longer life. Both studies found that death from all causes was reduced in study participants with weights that were 15 to 20 percent below the national average. In Okinawa, where adults and children are of lower body weight than in mainland Japan, the death rates from cardiovascular disease and cancer are lower by 30 to 40 percent.[12]

The reduction of 30 to 50 percent of the calories in the diet is an active area of research in both animal and human studies. The area of caloric restriction is extremely promising. Studies in animals have been positive and indicate that by reducing calories age is prolonged. Not only do the animals live longer than animals not calorically restricted but also they avoid diseases that are common causes of death. Lab animals develop heart disease and cancer, just as we humans do. But when lab animals are calorie restricted, they do not develop these conditions; instead, they simply "die" after a long life. It does not seem to matter when the caloric restriction is started. If animals are started with caloric restriction early in life, the onset of maturity is delayed and life span is increased. If the animals are started on caloric restriction after reaching maturity (adulthood), life span is increased.

Calorie-restricted animals have enhanced body chemistry. The cholesterol profile is improved. The markers of chronic inflammation in the body are reduced. The sensitivity to insulin increases. Intra-abdominal fat decreases. But underlying the chemical changes is a decrease in the production of reactive oxygen species (ROS) that characterize aging. Because caloric restriction lowers the rate of glycation, aging from this mechanism is eliminated. In effect, by giving the animals fewer calories it is possible to prevent disease, to prevent aging, and to extend their lives!

Studies in humans take longer to complete, because of our longer life span. But data from rhesus monkeys, closer to us on the evolutionary pyramid, have yielded the same data as other species studied. It is reasonable to believe that restricting calories will prevent diseases such as diabetes, cardiovascular disease, and cancers. In fact, these civilization-driven conditions appear to be caused by excessive calories!

One interesting experiment in caloric restriction in humans occurred by accident in the Biosphere 2 project. Biosphere 2 was a self-contained ecosystem mimicking the atmosphere of the Earth. On September 21, 1991, four men and four women were sealed into a structure in the Arizona desert that took in sunlight but was otherwise closed off from the rest of the world. Air, water, and organic material were recycled, and the participants grew their own food. But problems with producing sufficient food forced the Biospherians to limit their intake of food. The participants consumed vegetables, $\frac{1}{2}$ glass of milk daily, and meat once per week.

All eight lost weight: The men lost about 16 percent of their body weight, and the women about 11 percent. Their blood pressure was reduced, cholesterol dropped, and fasting glucose fell. The diet consumed in Biosphere 2 could have had a life-prolonging effect. Due to an unforeseen development, we were able to observe the effect of caloric restriction in humans for a short time. It would seem that the Biospherians benefited from a pure, unprocessed diet that was 30 percent lower in calories than normal.

DR. KLAUER'S CAVEATS FOR CALORIC RESTRICTION

1. Adequate nutrition must be maintained. If calories are restricted without adequate nutrition, you will become ill. Protein and calcium intakes must be optimal, or muscle and bone mass will suffer. Muscle wasting and osteoporosis are serious conditions resulting from too little protein and calcium. Follow your doctor's advice; you may not be a candidate for severe caloric restriction.
2. Expect to be cold. Caloric restriction causes body temperature to drop.
3. Don't attempt severe caloric restriction if you have had an abnormal EKG. It is safe for you to follow my diet plan, but not safe for you to limit your calories to the extent required by the severe caloric restriction plan.
4. Caloric restriction is not intended for children. During childhood, the body needs to grow and develop. Optimal height will not be achieved and mental development may be affected by too few calories.

People with a family history of age-related neurodegenerative disease may have a sense of a time bomb within them. Hereditary neurodegenerative diseases have a specific age of onset. Caloric restriction could potentially delay the onset of symptoms. By slowing down the aging process, caloric restriction may offer benefit to these people. Most of these diseases have no known cure; caloric restriction has the potential of adding years of quality life for people so afflicted.

This diet provides you with a life-enhancing and life-extending program. Chances are, you do not have the intention of moving to Okinawa or severely limiting your calories, but you know you need to make some meaningful improvements. Living a life of overconsumption and underactivity is a sure way to look older fast! This is exactly what most people do. Then they spend a fortune on cosmetics and spas, which do little to address the real problem. Sure, it feels great to put on a great-smelling cream or spend a week being pampered, but these do not address aging at a cellular level. To slow down the aging process requires more than just superficial changes. It requires eating the right foods, managing stress, and exercising regularly.

Chapter Eight

YOUR OUTSIDE IS A
MIRROR OF YOUR INSIDE

The right diet directs sexual energy into the parts that matter.

—DAME BARBARA CARTLAND

Youth is something very new. Twenty years ago, no one mentioned it. Nature gives you the face you have at twenty, it is up to you to merit the face you have at fifty.

—COCO CHANEL

• • •

High stress levels are a frequent complaint of my patients. That stress is associated with life in the big city is not new. But stress is also part of the life of a soccer mom in Duluth who is chauffeuring four children and managing a household, the Iowa farmer whose livelihood and crops are dependent on the amount of rainfall during growing season, and the eleventh-grade high school student concerned about college admission. In fact, stress has been with us since prehistoric times, when we had to worry about escaping the saber-toothed tiger. Stress has always been around and it always will be. It is part of life.

The "S" Word

The mind exerts a strong and powerful influence upon the body. Not only can the mind propel the body to perform superhuman feats of strength during times of stress but also our overall mental attitude affects our life expectancy. Depression decreases life expectancy and an optimistic attitude increases life span. Risk for disease is lower in people with a positive attitude on life.

Why this is so has to do with the presence of stress hormones in the body. Stress hormones are the "fight-or-flight hormones" named epinephrine, norepinephrine, and cortisol. These stress hormones helped us to run from hungry animals in prehistoric times by increasing our heart rate, blood pressure, and general alertness.

Today when we perceive danger these hormones have the same effect. While in prehistoric times, the fight-or-flight response was adaptive and related to real physical danger, now these powerful hormones are activated when there is no physical danger present but we feel threatened emotionally. This complicated chemical-emotional relationship has positive and negative implications for us. On the positive side, stress is not always *bad*; it can cause us to give our best performances and spur us on to excellence. Olympic athletes face enormous stress during competition, but this is how world records are set! When we have deadlines at work or must give presentations in front of groups, stress hormones can give us a competitive edge to work harder and to speak convincingly. But when stress is constant, it can have negative consequences for us. Chronic stress can shorten our lives.

The Effect of Stress on the Body

Stress and Reproduction

Cortisol reduces the amount of estrogen and testosterone produced, and inhibits the release of another hormone, lutenizing hormone or LH, which causes ovulation and sperm release. Females under excessive stress are known to have irregular periods because of this interaction.

Males will have lower sperm counts when chronically stressed. Couples with high levels of stress in their lives may find it difficult to conceive a baby because of this hormone.

When stress is high, sex drive is low. While prehistorically a low sex drive in times of stress was helpful and allowed for concentration to be directed at the source of danger, today it eliminates a potential stress fighter!

The Immune System and Stress

Cortisol lowers the body's ability to fight infection. It limits the body's ability to produce antibodies, which fight disease. Chronic stress lowers the white blood cell count, reducing our defense against illnesses. When we are stressed we are less able to fight off infection and are vulnerable to viruses, such as those that cause the flu and colds. High states of stress are equivalent to immunosuppression. The normal immune response is suppressed. In evolutionary terms, this evolved because, by concentrating all the body's energy into the stress response and not wasting it on the production of antibodies, the caveman escaped the immediate danger he faced and survived. Today, however, chronic stress is a *detriment* to our survival! Stress that is frequent or unabated keeps the body on "red alert," putting disease fighting on the back burner. We easily become ill and, when we do, because our disease fighting mechanism is impaired, recovery is slow.

Interestingly, the treatment of autoimmune diseases, which are states of excessive amounts of antibodies, involves corticosteroids, a class of drugs, that suppress the immune response. These drugs mimic cortisol's action on the immune system and dampen the overactive immune system.

Stress and Growth

Stress reduces the amount of growth hormone produced by the body as well as decreasing the response to insulin-like growth factor 1 (IGF-1). Premature infants are at risk for stunted growth. The stress of premature delivery and hospitalization results in production of high cortisol levels, retarding normal growth.

In adults, growth hormone and IGF-1 have the effect of increasing lean muscle mass, skin thickness, and improving memory. These hormones decline as we age. Chronic stress, by producing cortisol, lowers our natural levels of growth hormone and IGF-1 ahead of time. Although our body weight may not change, our muscle mass will decrease and fat mass will increase. Our body becomes flabby. Stress destroys the natural mechanism of cell renewal in our skin, causing dullness and sagging. In this case, excessive stress can have exactly the same effect upon the body as aging. Chronic stress can make us appear old and tired.

Stress and the Mind

Stress has been shown to impair memory. The system of the brain that governs short-term memory is weakened in stressful situations in which the individual has no control. The stress response increases our awareness of the environment. Vigilance is heightened but, if attention is not focused, distractibility is high. People taking an exam or reluctantly going onstage are familiar with this type of stress. The deterring factor here is *perceived* loss of control; when an individual is confident, although stressed, memory is unimpeded.

It should not come as a surprise to anyone that depression is related to stress. Chronic stress turns on the fight-or-flight response but doesn't turn it off again. The result is anxiety and overstimulation. Because this unpleasant state is unremitting, the individual feels helpless and hopeless. The excessive amount of cortisol produced in patients is responsible for the observed symptoms of depression. Disturbances of sleep, sexual function, and appetite are hallmarks of excess cortisol production.

Stress and Cardiovascular Disease

Chronic stress, by causing an increase in blood pressure, increases the risk for cardiovascular disease (heart attack and stroke). High stress levels cause the adrenal gland to produce more cortisol, which elevates body insulin. Excessive insulin causes visceral fat storage, an independent risk factor for type 2 diabetes and cardiovascular disease.

HOW STRESSED ARE YOU?

1. Have you gained or lost more than 5 pounds within the last year unintentionally?
2. Do you have trouble falling asleep? Do you wake during the night and have difficulty going back to sleep?
3. Is it difficult to concentrate on reading material? Are you casily distracted and forget what you were previously reading?
4. Do you have feelings of being overwhelmed? Is everything just "too much"?
5. Are you uninterested in sex?
6. Do you have a lack of energy? Are you tired all the time?
7. Are your palms cold and sweaty? Are you shaky?
8. Do you get frequent colds?
9. Are you becoming forgetful? Do you misplace your keys? Do you leave the headlights of your car on?
10. Have you recently had a major life change, such as a death, divorce, or job change?

If you answered yes to more than two or three of the above questions, stress is having a harmful effect on your health and putting you at risk. The levels of stress hormones are too high in your body and are causing physical symptoms.

Stress and Distress

Unquestionably, stress is part of life. To live in the modern world means a constant barrage of stressful stimuli; this is especially true in any urban setting, and particularly in New York City. It is also an important aspect of the Park Avenue mind-set. We are always rushing, running from place to place, and there are never enough hours in the day to get everything done. When traveling in the South or the UK, where time has a life of its own, most New Yorkers will lament that everyone moves so slowly.

An act as simple as trying to hail a taxi in the rain during rush hour causes acute stress for many Manhattanites. One must wait in line for movies and sporting events, and to enter cultural events. Museums offer wonderful shows but the more popular the show, the bigger the crowds that will attend. Often it is a challenge to view a work of art due to the large crowds. A feeling of stress and frustration develops in such situations as these. (I don't think there is an individual alive—aside from the Dalai Lama—who doesn't feel stressed hailing a cab in the rain or visiting an overcrowded museum exhibit.)

However, the appeal of New York City is its energy and liveliness. Sure, there is stress here, but people can learn to cope with it. For them, the good far outweighs the bad.

That is the attitude you need to have. It is not the stress itself but your reaction to it that determines whether you will be stimulated or "a stress victim."

There has been a constellation of personality traits described that seem to define a "stress-resistant personality."[1] These people seem to have attitudes and behaviors that help them to cope with stress efficiently. Stress-resistant people have an optimistic outlook on life, an internal sense of control, high levels of adaptability, and low levels of negative emotions (depression, hopelessness, hostility, and poor self-image). In short, they see themselves as achievers because they *are*! They have what I like to call a "fun and positive" attitude. Others are instinctively drawn to such people. It is not that these happy people have less stress in their lives; in fact, they often have high positions of responsibility, but *they cope with it better*. You can learn to respond to stress in a positive manner, if you do not already do so. It is essential that you master this.

The mind-body connection is a powerful one; let it work for your health and not against it!

ARE YOU STRESS RESISTANT?

1. Do you sleep well?
2. Have you maintained your weight in a normal range for a long period of time?
3. Do you feel "everything all works out in the end"?
4. Do you have many friends?
5. Do you enjoy meeting new people?
6. Do you laugh frequently?
7. Do you feel in control of your life? Of your emotions?
8. Have you received more than one invitation in the last month?
9. Are you happy?
10. Do you have a mutually rewarding relationship with a significant other?

The more times that you answered yes to the above questions, the more stress resistant you are. A score of less than 8 means you need to work on reducing stress. A score of 10 means you are invited to my next party!

Controlling the Stress Response

The techniques for managing stress are basically grouped into three categories: long-term strategies, short-term techniques, and mental-focus techniques. Each component is important, as each attacks a separate issue.

Long-Term Strategies

Long-term strategies are a matter of arranging your life so that your body is in top form. These are the things that are basic and nonnegotiable. Your life's pattern should be built around three elements:

1. *Exercise.* You must exercise. Daily. As discussed in chapter 6, exercise reduces stress by causing an outpouring of brain chemicals

called endorphins. Endorphins elevate mood and promote relaxation. (Endorphins have the exact opposite function of stress hormones.) Also, exercise causes the breakdown of fat, which necessitates release of free L-tryptophan. L-tryptophan is the precursor molecule of the "feel good" neurotransmitter, serotonin. Strong evidence exists for the efficacy of exercise in treating clinical depression. Additionally, exercise reduces anxiety and improves physical self-perceptions. We feel good and think we look good after a workout! Now, top psychiatrists recommend that patients commit to a regular schedule of physical exercise. Both aerobic and resistance exercise are associated with enhanced mood states.

2. *Diet.* Diet, too, can counter the negative aspects of stress. Eating on the run and eating high amounts of simple carbohydrates will amplify stress. Often, people who are stressed will turn to simple carbohydrates in an attempt to give themselves a boost of energy. This doesn't work. Fresh food, free of preservatives, will enable your body to perform its best. Protein helps to rebuild tissue damage; vegetables and fruits are sources of fiber and vital vitamins and minerals. Dairy products contain L-tryptophan, which helps raise serotonin levels. Fish and fish oil supplements have high omega-3 fat, and studies show that omega-3 fights the damage of stress. Omega-3 lowers the risk for heart attack, improves depression, and even makes the skin look better. My diet plan is the solution! It is vital to eat well when stress is present.

3. *Sleep.* Sleep is fundamental to health. Too little sleep is perceived by the body as a chronic stress state, causing the release of toxic stress hormones. Studies have shown the need for about 7 hours of sleep per night. There have been, and are, of course, extraordinary people who get by with less: Benjamin Franklin and Martha Stewart. But it is folly to think that by cutting back on your sleep you will match the achievements of either of these people!

The Connection Between Weight and Sleep

Production of leptin and ghrelin is influenced by how much or how little we sleep. Leptin and growth hormone rise to their peak during sleep so, when you are restricting your shut-eye, you are not allowing these important hormones to function properly. Leptin is the hormone that gives the brain information as to the adequacy of the body's energy stores. If you are not receiving that signal, your brain does not know that you have that energy available, so it seeks a source of energy in the form of easily digested carbohydrates—and increases your hunger. Have you ever experienced a sleepless night followed by a day when no matter what you ate you never felt satisfied?

How Hormones Affect Your Sleep

Leptin and ghrelin work in a kind of "checks and balances" system to control feelings of hunger and fullness. Leptin is a hormone produced by the fat cell that communicates to the brain how much energy (fat) the body has stored. The amount of leptin produced by the fat cell is dependent on the amount of fat within the fat cell, so a large fat cell will produce a high amount of leptin. Likewise, a heavy person will have a higher level of leptin than someone who is slim. When we go on a diet, our fat cells shrink and leptin levels fall, causing a stronger hunger drive, a direct result of the brain sensing a lower level of leptin. In evolutionary terms, this stronger hunger drive was a survival mechanism that pushed us to search for food during times of famine. Lower leptin also causes us to conserve energy.

Ghrelin is a hormone produced in the stomach that signals hunger to the brain. So what's the connection to sleep? Leptin levels have a circadian rhythm, which means they are highest during sleep. When you don't get enough sleep, peak leptin levels are not reached, which the brain interprets as reduced energy stores. You feel hungry. You don't want to be as active. Lack of sleep also causes ghrelin levels to rise, which means your appetite is stimulated; in other words, you want more food. The two combined can set the stage for overeating, which in turn may lead to weight gain.

Those Who Sleep Less Often Weigh More

How the hormones leptin and ghrelin set the stage for overeating was recently explored in two studies conducted at the University of Chicago in Illinois and at Stanford University in California.

In the Chicago study, doctors measured levels of leptin and ghrelin in twelve healthy men. The doctors also noted hunger and appetite levels. Soon after, the men were subjected to two days of sleep deprivation followed by two days of extended sleep. During this time doctors continued to monitor hormone levels, appetite, and activity.

The end result: When sleep was restricted, leptin levels went down and ghrelin levels went up. Not surprisingly, the men's appetite also increased proportionally. Their desire for high-carbohydrate, calorie-dense foods increased by a whopping 45 percent.

In a joint project between Stanford and the University of Wisconsin, about one thousand volunteers reported the number of hours they slept each night. Doctors then measured their levels of ghrelin and leptin, as well as charted their weight. Those who slept less than 8 hours a night not only had lower levels of leptin and higher levels of ghrelin, but they also had a higher level of body fat. What's more, that level of body fat seemed to correlate with their sleep patterns. Specifically, those who slept the fewest hours per night weighed the most.

If you are trying to lose weight, when you log in a few extra hours of sleep a week, you may discover that you aren't as hungry, or that you have lessened your craving for sugary, calorie-dense foods. Once people are not as tired, they don't need to rely on sweet foods and high-carbohydrate snacks to keep them awake, which translates into eating fewer calories.

Sleep Apnea

Physical abnormalities inside the mouth and neck cause the soft tissue in the rear of the throat to collapse. This briefly closes off air passages many times during a night, causing disruption in breathing, called "sleep apnea," and a tendency to snore. So although you may go to bed early and think you are getting a good night's rest, sleep apnea prevents you from experiencing a deep sleep. Eight hours of disrupted sleep can leave you feeling like you had only 4. You wake up feeling tired and continue to feel tired all day.

I have had patients who, when successfully treated for their weight, had their sleep apnea resolve. As they lost the weight, they slept better and had more energy, so they were more active and just ate less.

The Stages of Sleep

We actually fall asleep in stages. When our head first hits the pillow, we close our eyes, and we get into a comfortable position, we are said to be in stage 1 of sleep. During stage 2 sleep we are in "light sleep" and are easily aroused. The most restorative stages are during deep sleep, stages 3 and 4. In deep sleep, our muscles are completely relaxed, our heartbeat and respiratory rates slowed. It is during deep sleep that muscle repair takes place and growth hormone is released. The period of sleep with rapid eye movement, REM sleep, is when we dream. It is postulated that REM sleep allows the mind to relax and regain creativity. The normal sleep pattern has approximately four or five cycles of REM sleep but, when sleep is disordered, there is less time asleep and less time spent in deep sleep and in REM sleep.[2] The result is less benefit from the act of sleep and from a lower amount of growth hormone released. Disordered sleep is marked by a longer time to fall asleep, nightmares and anxiety dreams, excessive movement of the legs during sleep, awakening during the night, and inability to fall asleep again. In attempting to fall asleep people worry that sleep will not occur, and the desire for sleep itself becomes a stressor. The harder you try to sleep, the more difficult it becomes.

On the Klauer Plan, there are specific techniques that will enable you to make restorative and sound sleep part of your life. Once you have mastered these concepts they become automatic, even if you have had years of restless sleep. It is all just a matter of habit. Your life becomes balanced. Sleep techniques are ways of allowing your body to naturally relax and fall asleep.

Bill is a fifty-year-old investment banker with a long history of sleep problems. He goes to sleep just fine but wakes and worries about the stock market and his business. He was able to let go of this long-standing pattern by two simple measures: (1) He kept a pad on his night table, on which he wrote down important business insights that occurred to him prior to sleep. By writing them down, he was relieved of the stress that he might forget these details. Once the ideas were committed to paper, he could relax. (2) He practiced progressive relaxation, consciously relaxing each muscle group. As he relaxed, he focused on all he had to be thankful for. Like the old song, he "counted his blessings instead of sheep, he fell asleep counting his blessings." His sleep was restored fully within 2 weeks. As an aside, an added benefit is that Bill has become even more successful at work and is happier in his personal life. He controls his stress, rather than the other way around.

RESTORATIVE SLEEP TECHNIQUES

- Drink a glass of warm milk. Remember how your mother told you to do this? Once again, Mom had it right. There are proteins in milk that may act as a natural sedative. Lactose intolerant? Try a cup of yogurt.
- Check through the list provided in this book to see if medications that you are taking might be interfering with sleep. There are many common medications that interfere with sleep and sometimes physicians forget to mention insomnia as a side effect.
- Establish a deadline of 7:00 P.M. for having anxiety-provoking discussions. Never start an argument before bedtime. Going to bed angry harms any relationship and negatively affects your sleep and health.
- Have a ritual that you follow before sleep. Take your bath or shower. Lavender is an herb that naturally induces sleep; the benefit of this was shown in a clinical trial of elderly people. When they were each given a small bag of lavender to put under their pillow, sleep occurred faster and was perceived as more restful. Use a lavender-scented body lotion or have a small lavender sachet by your pillow. Its lovely scent will calm you.
- Reserve your bed just for sleep and sex. Do your reading sitting in a chair. Never watch TV in bed.
- After you have turned off the light, allow yourself to progressively relax each muscle in your body, beginning with your forehead. Focus on how perfectly formed your body is, and be thankful for the day that you have just experienced.

COMMON PRESCRIPTION DRUGS KNOWN TO CAUSE INSOMNIA[3]

Antihypertensives

Clonidine
Beta-blockers: Propanolol, Atenolol, Pindolol
Reserpine

Hormones

Oral contraceptives   Cortisone
Thyroid preparations   Progesterone

Sympathomimetic Amines

Bronchodilators: Tarbutaline, Apounduterol, Salmeterol, Metapro-
  terenol
Xanthine derivatives: Theophylline
Decongestants: Phenylpropanolamine, Pseudoephedrine

Antineoplastics
Miscellaneous

Phenytoin   Levodopa
Nicotine   Quinidine

Hidden Caffeine

Caffeine can be found in many things other than just coffee and
chocolate. It is present in over-the-counter products such as
Anacin, Excedrin, Empirin, and cough and cold preparations.

Short-Term Techniques

Even if you have a perfectly healthy lifestyle, there will undoubtedly come a time when you are taken by surprise by a stressful situation. It is just the way life is.

These techniques can help:

- Studies have shown a very interesting difference between men and women, in regard to a stressful situation. When women are exposed to stress, they tend to hold their breath. You can often hear this in their voices: Their voice goes up an octave or two. With men, this is not the case. Breath-holding has an effect within the body of raising CO_2, which causes blood pressure to rise. This is important because elevated blood pressure is harmful to the heart. If you are a woman and you are in a stressful situation, concentrate on your breathing. Take a few deep breaths, breathing deeply as you inhale; hold for a second or two, and exhale thoroughly. Be aware of your breathing and your voice quality; these are linked, as any voice coach will tell you.

- Act, don't react. Many unpleasant situations are preceded by warning signals that we choose to ignore. This form of denial does nothing but allow the situation to fester. Don't sweep it under the rug! Get everything out into the open. By speaking up early you set the tone and you can think over what you need to communicate. Your message is thoughtful and you make your concerns known. Communication should be assertive and not abusive. Imagine yourself in the other individuals' position and how you would like to be spoken to (other than just being told you are "the greatest"). Make your criticism constructive. Mix praise with criticism. Let individuals know what they are doing well but how they can improve. This is what will get you the results that you want.

- If a situation is just too much for you, walk away. There is nothing wrong with taking a breather. I think it is better to do this than to say things that you may regret later. Take a walk around the block, get on the treadmill, or go to the gym. Physical exertion relieves the emotional stress. You will raise mood-elevating endorphins. This is not to be confused with avoidance. Be mindful that the reprieve is only temporary; when you return, address the issue head on!

- During a stressful day, try to stretch. It doesn't matter if you only have 15 seconds. Do some neck and shoulder rolls; we tend to feel stress here. Stretching will help. Besides relieving the muscle tension, a stretch also takes the focus away from the situation and onto our health.
- Never eat out of stress. You will just feel worse because of the inevitable crash following a sugar high. Make sure there are healthy snacks handy, not empty calories in the form of processed foods. The stress is only temporary and you do not want to be left with a souvenir of weight gain to remember it by. The more times you can get through stressful times without pacifying yourself with food, the easier it becomes.

COMBAT STRESS

- Act, don't react.
- Concentrate on breathing.
- Stretch.
- Don't reach for food.
- Take a timeout.

Mental-Focus Techniques

Generalized anxiety disorder is the most common psychiatric disorder in the United States, aside from substance abuse.[4] It is marked by difficulty sleeping, excessive worrying, fatigue, and muscle tension. It is commonly precipitated by stress. The excess levels of stress hormones can increase the risk for panic attacks, alcohol abuse, and major depression.[5] Anxiety's high hormonal stress levels would seem to be harmful to the brain chemistry as well as body chemistry.

The mind can be controlled and anxiety relieved through the power of meditation. The efficacy of the mind in controlling the body is thousands of years old. Tibetan monks are able to slow their heart rates to extremely low levels. Indeed, biofeedback is used to reduce blood pressure after a heart attack. What about using biofeedback to maintain health before getting sick? What about allowing our minds to protect us against mental and physical illness? It is not only possible but essential.

Mind over Matter

We are all acquainted with mental-focus techniques: listening intently to music, studying for exams, and so on. Did you know that prayer may also be considered a mental-focus technique? By focusing us on a higher being, prayer allows us to direct our minds away from the day's hectic pace and concentrate on what matters. When we pray, we become aware of the smallness of our worries within the infinity of creation. We reflect on who we are and how precious life is. The common thread in prayers of all religions is the greatness of the Creator and thankfulness for our lives.

Also, regular meditation has been shown to increase the brain's ability to learn and improve memory. The brain's activity is composed of bursts of electrical activity of various waveforms. Each different waveform is characteristic of a mental state; for example, alpha waves predominate during daydreaming and drowsiness. On the other hand, gamma waves are characteristic of focused concentration, when we are completely involved in a mental pursuit. A recent comparison study of Buddhist monks who had each spent over ten thousand hours in meditation, and novice meditators found that both groups showed increased brain gamma waves during meditation.[6] While the monks had a high increase in gamma waves and showed a higher level of these waves at baseline, the novice meditators were able to increase their gamma waves during meditation as they became more adept. The fact that there was an increase in ability to focus attention is significant. It means that we should be able to induce this change within ourselves. Even more significant was that the elevation in gamma waves persists even without being in the meditative state. By spending time mediating daily, our baseline ability to concentrate and to focus is increased. Even when we are not meditating, we are more alert and attuned to the moment. Another way to describe this is "mindfulness" and "being in the moment." This translates to focused concentration; we do not worry about the past or present, we are involved in what is happening now.

Another form of mental focus is self-hypnosis. In my clinical practice, I encourage my patients to use hypnosis to become self-aware. Hypnosis has been given a bad name by pseudohypnotists who encourage patrons to "bark like a dog" or other ridiculous antics. The fact is that no one does anything that he or she do not want to do under hypnosis. Hypnosis is a state of focused awareness. By this I mean, as you are reading this paragraph, you are also aware of your surroundings. You can be said to have "peripheral concentration." You are aware of your children in the next room and the peach-colored upholstery of the chair in which you sit. But if you have ever experienced the sensation of driving down a highway and becoming mesmerized by the road ahead or if you have ever become so engrossed in a book you were reading that you became unaware of your surroundings, then you have experienced a state of "focused concentration." You have experienced a trance state!

Athletes are very familiar with this state; it is called "being in the zone." In the zone, they are focused entirely upon the game. They don't worry about their opponent or whether they have the ability to win. They concentrate *entirely* on the ball. They become formidable competitors because of their ability to become totally absorbed in what they are doing. Olympic medals are won because of focused concentration!

You need not be an Olympic athlete or performer to experience a focused concentration. If you allow yourself to achieve a high degree of concentration in any task, you can do it masterfully. Why not begin with your health? Take time to center your mind and meditate on how to care for yourself. This will bring awareness toward a healthier life.

Achieving Focused Concentration
To enter a state of focused concentration, you must be free from distraction. Your environment should be calm and peaceful. Sit or lie in a comfortable position wearing garments that do not constrict your body. Turn off the telephone ringer. Nothing must interrupt you. This time is just for YOU.

Pick a mental image of yourself—such as how great you will look at your goal weight. Or if a challenging situation is approaching, you can imagine the specific techniques that you will use to triumph. The image should be personal and pertinent to what you want to accomplish; the important point is to make the image as specific and as detailed as possible.

The image is a picture to guide you. Often, as you lose a lot of weight, you can have a sense that your body doesn't belong to you. A feeling of being disconnected to your body and a sense of unreality can cause a relapse, just to get back to a place of familiarity. The more weight that is lost, the greater the risk for dissociation. Seeing a different body than the one that has become familiar can be unsettling. Do not allow your serious efforts to be thwarted by an unprepared emotional state. Give yourself the advantage of preparing mentally; it is the difference between success and failure. You must become comfortable with your slim, trim body before achieving it. By doing so, you are giving yourself a guarantee that the change is permanent.

Start thinking of yourself as a thin person!

SELF-HYPNOSIS

Below is an exercise that I use to teach my patients to achieve a focused relaxed state. It is what I say to help them achieve this state. I offer it here in an effort to give you a technique for complete relaxation.

Begin by taking a deep breath, allowing your lungs to completely fill with air. Hold for a second or two and then exhale, while allowing yourself to relax very deeply. Again inhale and hold for a second or two and then exhale, allowing tension to leave your body. For the third breath, breathe in deeply, becoming aware of your lungs filling with life-giving oxygen. This time while you exhale, truly allow all stress to leave your body. Tell yourself, "Good. Now I am in a place of safety and relaxation. I am at peace. I feel no tension." Now be aware of the muscles of your forehead: Are they holding tension? If so, just let it go. Relax. Become aware of the muscles of your neck and shoulders. Are you aware of any tension being held in this area? Relax. Focus on the muscles of your biceps and triceps; relax them. Relax your hands; focus on them as they rest by your sides or in your lap. They are not holding stress, the fingers are not clenched but

(continued)

in a relaxed state, as your entire body is becoming more and more at peace and calm. Again, inhale deeply and let it go. While exhaling, be mindful of the tranquility that you now feel. Good. Feel your thighs pressing against the chair in which you are sitting; let go of tension in your hamstrings and your quadriceps. These strong muscles are at rest; just as they enable your body to walk and run during the day, now they must let go of stress. Take another deep breath and exhale. Last, feel your feet and your toes resting on the floor and let any tension held there leave your body. Your entire body and mental state is now in a state of deep relaxation. You are not asleep because you are conscious of your body's sensations.

Now imagine a beautiful place that pleases you. The air is pure, the temperature is mild. It is a beautiful, peaceful day. Picture a crystal clear lake. The water is just the right temperature. Imagine yourself floating on the pure and pleasant water. The water gently caresses your body. Imagine how it feels on your back, your head, and your arms and legs. It supports your body. Now visualize your body, slim and healthy. Your body is strong. Your body is perfect. It is perfect as the water that supports it. Your body is wondrous.

As you calmly and peacefully float in the pure water, visualize your internal organs. They are amazingly formed. Your lungs bring oxygen from the environment into your body. Your heart beats effortlessly throughout your life, without you even being aware of it. Your heart's strong contractions cause oxygen to be carried to all the cells of your body. These life processes occur effortlessly and without thought on your part. Visualize your digestive system, which allows nourishment from food to enter your body. The process of life is a marvel. You are the caretaker of this incredible vessel.

Just as you might guide a small child while crossing the street, looking in both directions for approaching cars, you might even caution the child about the danger of the intersec-

(continued)

tion. So, too, you must cautiously guard and protect your own perfect body against harm.

Tell yourself that your body is a gift that you must take care of. Overeating is a poison. You must only give yourself foods that will protect and honor your body. Visualize your body as you see yourself floating peacefully. Visualize your arms and legs, strong and without excessive fat. See your waist slim and defined. Your body is meant to be slim and sleek. You will return to the body you are meant to have.

Now visualize yourself emerging from the water, happy and refreshed. Notice how gracefully your body moves. You feel light and you are confident. You are aware of your power to affect your own health. Repeat again to yourself, "My body is a wondrous gift. I must protect it. Overeating is a poison. I will not poison my body."

As you ready yourself to leave the trance state, remind yourself to stay focused on the resolutions that you have made. You will achieve them. Your goal is a worthy one. You will achieve it. You will protect your body. Your body is slim and healthy. Inhale deeply and as you exhale, open your eyes. You are resolved. You are confident. You will achieve your goal.

The practice of self-hypnosis is part of the plan to guide you toward overall health. There are temptations and distractions that conspire to lure your attention away from your goal of weight loss and health. You must coach yourself from the other side. Self-hypnosis will keep you focused on the magnificence of your body. Just as you would not fill a Mercedes with cheap gasoline, so you must not fill your incredible body with poor-quality food! By taking the time to meditate on your body, you are increasing your armor against the disease- and age-promoting environment that surrounds you.

STRESS RELIEVERS

Sometimes you need immediate help in dealing with stress or tension. You do not have a full 15 minutes or even 5 minutes to devote to relaxation techniques. Try these:

1. *The Inner Smile.* Imagine someone dear to you. Recall the love that you feel toward this person. Imagine yourself smiling. Feel the muscles of your face beginning to form a smile. This is an extremely relaxing sensation, tension leaves the face. As you engage your smile muscles, breathe in deeply. As you exhale, imagine all tension leaving your body. Concentrate on your loved one and the inner smile. How happy you are to see the person, feel the smile. Complete the sequence for several times.

2. *15-Second Breather.* Inhale slowly and deeply for a count of 5. Then exhale completely for a count of 5. As you inhale say to yourself, "one, two, three," and so on. Count backward as you exhale, "five, four, three," and so on. Repeat the sequence five times.

Do the stress-relieving exercises when you are put on hold on the telephone, stuck in traffic, standing in line, waiting in an airport, or feeling frustrated or annoyed. Or anytime.

In Conclusion

By using relaxation techniques, you remove stress from your body. Think for a moment of the faces of the Tibetan monks; they are serene and unlined. They do not have wrinkles or appear anxious. The monks are free of stress because of their focused concentration on the magnificence of creation. The people of Okinawa have the same radiation of happiness. Although your surroundings and culture may be very different from the Okinawans and Tibetans you, too, can achieve a higher state of serenity.

Use the principles that I have outlined, even if you don't believe that they will work. What do you have to lose? You may find, as many others have, they are valuable tools against stress.

Think about food in terms of nutrition and energy, which is what it was intended for. People with weight issues too often see food as more important than it should be. Remember, food is not comfort, nor is it a method of coping. Changing how you think about food and its role in your life will help you think, and live, like a healthy person.

The Klauer Plan combines the best foods, daily exercise, and a set of stress-combating techniques. We all need to continually challenge our ways of thinking and living. If we are fortunate enough to have the sacred trust of good health, let us do everything to safeguard it. By living our lives thoughtfully and with exuberance, we can preserve our health. We are all capable of so much more than we think. Whether you live in New York City, Dallas, Anchorage, or Paris, the principles of proactive health apply. You will become younger looking and acting. You will transform your life as you transform your body. It's up to you to do it.

Chapter Nine

DR. KLAUER'S RECIPES

*People who eat white bread have no
dreams!*

—DIANA VREELAND

• • •

Just because you are restricting your calories does not mean that you
must eliminate the pleasure of eating. Indeed, eating is a pleasure that
can improve your health! It just depends upon what you consume.

It is a joy to savor the aroma of food cooking on the stove. Why not
allow yourself to experience the best foods? I believe Diana Vreeland
meant that a bland American diet of processed food is not only unhealthy,
but has no style!

Exuberance and experimentation in cooking are paramount to excellence. Fresh vegetables and herbs, filling and flavorful, are practi-
cally calorie free. There are creative menu solutions to every occasion.
Many of my patients have come up with some delicious ideas. These
recipes have enabled them to stay on the health path while losing
weight. I pass them along to you as a gift and encourage you to experiment. Bon appétit!

The Right to Dine: Starters, Snacks, and Dressings

A sprinkle of caviar is an ideal accompaniment to an omelet, or use it as a garnish on various dishes, to add a touch of glamour. Caviar adds taste, texture, and elegance to a dish, and is a rich source of omega-3 fats. One ounce has only 70 calories.

THE TSARINA'S OYSTER AND CAVIAR MARTINI

1/2 cup minced shallots
4 tablespoons chopped fresh dill
1/4 cup champagne vinegar
Juice of fresh lemon
2 tablespoons fresh, coarsely ground black pepper
36 oysters in shell
Crushed ice
2 ounces (60 grams) Beluga caviar

1. In a small bowl, mix the shallots, dill, vinegar, lemon juice, and ground pepper.
2. Shuck the oysters and with sharp knife separate the muscles from the shell.
3. Fill a large, wide-mouthed martini glass with crushed ice, then arrange the oyster shells on top with oysters replaced in shell. Spoon the sauce over the oysters and top with a dollop of caviar.

SERVING SIZE: 3 OYSTERS • CALORIES: 25 • PROTEIN: 2 G • FAT: 1.5 G •
SODIUM: 85 G

CAPRESE SALAD

Made with fresh part-skim mozzarella that can be found at specialty cheese purveyors, such as Grace's Marketplace, this dish is sure to please. It is my husband's favorite summer salad.

Large, fresh basil leaves
2 to 3 ripe organic beefsteak tomatoes
1 large red onion, thinly sliced
8 ounces part-skim fresh mozzarella, sliced evenly
Balsamic vinegar

1. Lay the basil leaves in a pinwheel formation on a serving plate.
2. Arrange the tomato sheet, onion slices, and mozzarella sheet alternately, in a circle on the basil leaves.
3. Drizzle with balsamic vinegar.

SERVES 4 • SERVING SIZE: 186 G • CALORIES: 203 • TOTAL FAT: 12 G • SAT FAT: 7 G • CHOL: 31 MG • SODIUM: 304 MG • CARBS: 10 G • FIBER: 2 G • SUGARS: 4 G • PROTEIN: 16 G

LENTIL SALAD WITH WALNUT AND ORANGE BALSAMIC DRESSING

1 cup dried French lentils
1/4 teaspoon iodized table salt
2 ounces freshly squeezed orange juice
2 tablespoons aged balsamic vinegar (see note)
1/2 tablespoon Dijon mustard
1/2 tablespoon extra-virgin olive oil
1/4 teaspoon ground black pepper
1/2 cup carrots, chopped
3 tablespoons chopped scallions
4 teaspoons chopped black walnuts*
4 cups spinach, well rinsed, trimmed, leaves chopped (leaves only)

*Black walnuts have a rich nutty texture, and are mainly used in baking because of their delicious, potent flavor.

1. In a saucepan, bring 3 cups of water to a boil over high heat.
2. Add the lentils and a pinch of salt, cook until lentils are tender but still hold their shape (about 25 minutes—do not overcook!). Then drain.
3. In a large mixing bowl, whisk together the orange juice, balsamic vinegar, mustard, olive oil, pepper, and the rest of the salt.
4. Stir in the drained lentils, carrots, scallions, and walnuts. Add the spinach, tossing to mix well.

SERVING SIZE: 2 CUPS • CALORIES: 256 • CALORIES FROM FAT: 67 • TOTAL FAT: 7.4 G • CHOL: 0 • CARBS: 34.2 G • PROTEIN: 16.1 G

Note: Good balsamic vinegar should have a robust and tangy taste that falls somewhere between sweet and sour. It can be served over flakes of Parmigiano-Reggiano cheese, sprinkled on a fresh salad; used as a glaze for steak, pork, or poultry; or drizzled over berries (see dessert menus).

TOMATO EDAMAME SALAD

1/2 pound green beans, cut into thirds and ends trimmed off
2 cups edamame, shelled
3 scallions, thinly sliced
1 pint cherry tomatoes, cut into halves
1 handful fresh basil, chopped
1 tablespoon rice vinegar
1 tablespoon fresh lime juice
1 teaspoon honey
1 teaspoon Dijon mustard
2 teaspoons olive oil
Dash of salt and freshly ground pepper to taste

1. In a steamer basket over lightly boiling water, cook the green beans and edamame until tender but crisp, approximately 5 minutes. Drain and set aside to cool.
2. Combine the scallions, tomatoes, basil, and cooked edamame and beans, tossing to mix.

3. In a small bowl, prepare a dressing with the vinegar, lime juice, honey, and mustard, whisking in the olive oil. Pour the dressing over the vegetables and toss to coat. This unusual combination of beans may be served chilled or at room temperature. Serves 6

SERVING SIZE: 65 G • CALORIES: 80 • TOTAL FAT: 6 G • SAT FAT: 1 G • CHOL: 0 • SODIUM: 6 MG • CARBS: 5 G • FIBER: 2 G • SUGARS: 1 G • PROTEIN: 4 G

TUSCAN WHITE BEAN AND SPINACH SOUP

2 cups dried cannellini white beans (rinsed and picked over)
6 cups water
1 teaspoon salt
1 bay leaf
2 tablespoons olive oil
1 yellow onion, coarsely chopped
6 cloves garlic, chopped
$1/4$ teaspoon freshly ground pepper
1 tablespoon chopped fresh rosemary
1 pound spinach, cooked and chopped
$1^1/_2$ cups vegetable or chicken stock

1. Soak the beans overnight and drain. (Soaking beans overnight prevents stomach gas.)
2. In a big soup pot, combine the beans, water, $1/2$ teaspoon of salt, and the bay leaf. Bring to a boil, then reduce to a simmer, partially covered, until the beans are tender, approximately 1 hour and 15 minutes.
3. Drain the beans, reserving $1/2$ cup of the liquid. Discard the bay leaf.
4. In a small bowl, combine the reserved cooking liquid and $1/2$ cup of the cooked beans. Mash with a fork. This will be used to thicken the soup. (I suggest this technique as a way of thickening both soups and sauces. Just mix a small amount of cooking liquid with a pureed vegetable or legume, and mix into the liquid portion of what you are cooking. It will replace the high-calorie and nutritionally deficient old method of forming a roux with butter, flour, and broth as a thickener.)
5. Return the pot to the stovetop and add the olive oil, onion, and garlic. Sauté these together until the onion is translucent.

6.   Stir in the remaining ¹/₂ teaspoon of salt, the pepper, and the rose-
      mary, spinach, bean mixture, and stock.

7.   Bring to a boil, then reduce to a simmer and allow to heat through-
      out and the flavors to blend, approximately 15 minutes. Ladle into
      soup bowls and enjoy! Serves 6.

SERVING SIZE: 277 G • CALORIES: 312 • TOTAL FAT: 6 G • SAT FAT: 1 G • CHOL:
0 • SODIUM: 364 MG • CARBS: 49 G • FIBER: 14 G • SUGARS: 3 G •
PROTEIN: 21 G

MISO SOUP

Miso soup is made from fermented soybeans. It is delicious and high
in protein. Tofu is also made from soybeans. The subtle Asian flavors
make this a protein-rich and delicious way to begin the meal.

1 clove garlic
3 scallions
1 tablespoon peeled and finely chopped fresh ginger
1 tablespoon olive oil
4 cups chicken or vegetable stock
2 tablespoons white miso
¹/₄ pound firm tofu, drained and cut into ¹/₄-inch cubes
3 ounces fresh shiitake mushrooms, thinly sliced
1 cup watercress leaves

1.   Sauté the garlic, scallions, and ginger in the olive oil together until
      translucent.

2.   Add the stock and bring to a boil. Reduce to a simmer.

3.   Whisk in the miso until dissolved. Add the tofu, mushrooms, and
      watercress, and simmer until the tofu is heated through and mush-
      rooms and watercress are softened.

4.   Ladle into small Asian-style soup bowls. Serves 6.

SERVING SIZE: 245 G • CALORIES: 91 • TOTAL FAT: 4 G • SAT FAT: 1 G •
CHOL: 0 • SODIUM: 1,166 MG • CARBS: 11 G • FIBER: 2 G • SUGARS: 3 G
• PROTEIN: 5 G

CARLA'S SALSA VERDE

This terrific recipe is from Carla, one of my patients who has a real flair for cooking! This is a spicy and delicious accompaniment to any type of fish.

It is made with tomatillos, which provide the tart flavor in Mexican green sauces. In Mexico they are also called *tomatoes verdes, tomates de cáscara*, as well as *fresadillas*.

5 tomatillos (remove the husks)
1/4 cup fresh cilantro
1 medium-size onion
1/2 jalapeño pepper

1. Boil the tomatillos until soft but not mushy. Drain.
2. In the food processor, chop the cilantro and onion.
3. Add the tomatillos and jalapeño pepper, and puree all the ingredients together.

SERVING SIZE: 298 G (ENTIRE RECIPE) • CALORIES: 106 • TOTAL FAT: 2 G • SAT FAT: 0 • CHOL: 0 • SODIUM: 7 MG • CARBS: 22 G • FIBER: 5 G • SUGARS: 22 G • PROTEIN: 3 G

RED AND GREEN GUACAMOLE DIP

This is a delicious accompaniment to fresh, crisp crudités, instead of tortilla chips that are loaded with salt and fat.

1 large avocado, halved and pitted
6 ounces "lite" silken tofu
1/2 cup chopped Italian tomatoes, seeds removed
1/4 cup diced red onion
1/2 cup chopped fresh cilantro
Juice of 1/2 large lime
1/4 teaspoon sea salt
1/2 teaspoon white pepper

1.   Place the avocado halves in a large bowl. Mash with a fork until no large pieces are remaining.
2.   Place the tofu in a food processor or blender, and process until smooth.
3.   Combine avocado and tofu, mixing well until thoroughly blended.
4.   Stir in remaining ingredients, mixing until blended.
5.   Refrigerate unused portion for up to 3 days.

SERVING SIZE: ¼ CUP • CALORIES: 65 • PROTEIN: 3 G • CALCIUM: 32 MG

GINGER SOY DRESSING

This tangy dressing may also be used for a marinade for shrimp, fish, chicken, or grilled tofu.

¼ cup Japanese wine vinegar
¼ teaspoon Thai roasted chile garlic paste (available in
    specialty markets)
2 teaspoons garlic, finely minced (1 to 2 cloves)
1 tablespoon thinly sliced scallions
2 teaspoons finely minced fresh ginger
1 cup unsweetened orange juice
¼ cup light soy sauce
1 teaspoon sugar

Blend all ingredients with a wire whisk and allow to chill thoroughly. Yield: 1½ cups.

SERVING SIZE: 1 TABLESPOON • CALORIES: 5 • FAT: 0 • CARBS: 1 G •
PROTEIN: 0.5 G

LIME-SHOYU VINAIGRETTE

⅓ cup fresh lime juice
¼ cup extra-virgin olive oil
2 tablespoons low-sodium soy sauce
2 tablespoons Dijon mustard

1. Mix all ingredients in a small jar and shake well.
2. Use immediately or refrigerate for up to 5 days.
3. Bring to room temperature and shake well before using.

SERVING SIZE: 2 TABLESPOONS • CALORIES: 89 • CALORIES FROM FAT: 84 •
TOTAL FAT: 9.4 G • CHOL: 0 • SODIUM: 240 MG • CARBS: 2.1 G • PROTEIN: 0.7 G

MUSTARD VINAIGRETTE

A wonderful light dressing for all sorts of fresh greens. This can also be brushed on chicken as marinade before grilling.

Juice of ½ fresh lemon
1 tablespoon red wine vinegar
1 teaspoon Dijon mustard
1 tablespoon first-press extra-virgin olive oil
Dash of salt
¼ teaspoon coarsely ground pepper

1. To make the vinaigrette, in a small bowl, whisk together lemon juice, vinegar, and mustard.
2. While whisking, slowly pour in the oil in a thin stream, allowing it to become gradually incorporated into the mix. Whisk in the salt and pepper.

SERVING SIZE: 11 G • CALORIES: 22 • TOTAL FAT: 2 G • SAT FAT: 0 • CHOL: 0
• SODIUM: 9 MG • CARBS: 1 G • FIBER: 0 • SUGARS: 0 • PROTEIN: 0

Note: Use the Mustard Vinaigrette when you toss your salad. If you would like to save a few calories, wash and spin salad greens, then toss the salad with dressing in a separate bowl, then put the dressed salad back into your salad spinner and spin again. The result is the leaves will be coated with dressing but excess is avoided!

CREAMY HERB DRESSING

$^1/_2$ cup Italian parsley, chopped
2 tablespoons chopped fresh dill
1 scallion
$^1/_2$ cup low-fat buttermilk
$^1/_2$ cup fat-free plain yogurt
1 garlic clove
1 tablespoon extra-virgin olive oil
Salt and pepper to taste

1. Chop herbs in the food processor until finely chopped. Add the remaining ingredients and process to combine.
2. Refrigerate until use.
3. Pour over salads or use as a dip.

SERVING SIZE: $^1/_4$ CUP   •   CALORIES: 49   •   TOTAL FAT: 3 G   •   SAT FAT: 0.53 G   •   CHOL: 1.35 MG   •   CARBS: 3 G   •   FIBER: 0.2 G   •   PROTEIN: 1.6 G   •   CALCIUM: 82 MG

PARMESAN CRISPS

These are delicious as a snack and also in salads as a healthy substitute for croutons. They are a great source of calcium and protein. For variety, you can add finely chopped fresh rosemary to the mixture.

Wedge of Parmesan cheese*
Olive oil to coat a baking sheet

*Parmesan is also known as Parmigiano-Reggiano. The traditional marking with the inscription in full, "Parmigiano-Reggiano," should be impressed along the side of the whole cheese, which should allow you to identify it even on small pieces. The name itself refers to the towns of Parma and Reggio Emilia, in Italy. The structure of the cheese is also unmistakable; it should be granular and break easily into slivers, with a fragrant and delicate aroma. It is known to have a high protein and vitamin content, and for its wealth of calcium and phosphorus.

1. Preheat oven to 350°F.
2. Grate the Parmesan cheese coarsely or with a food processor.
3. Shape the cheese into 1-inch-diameter balls, using a teaspoon. Drop the Parmesan balls onto a lightly oiled cooking sheet lined with parchment paper, spacing them about 3 inches apart.
4. Bake in middle of oven at 350°F until brown and bubbly. Watch closely, or they will burn! They should bake for approximately 5 minutes.
5. Remove carefully with a metal spatula. Cool on a plate and then store in airtight container for up to 1 week.

SERVING SIZE: 19 G • CALORIES: 92 • TOTAL FAT: 7 G • SAT FAT: 3 G • CHOL: 15 MG • SODIUM: 225 MG • CARBS: 1 G • FIBER: 0 • SUGARS: 0 • PROTEIN: 6 G

Hummus is often overlooked in a diet program. This Middle Eastern treat is a wonderfully satisfying and nutritious aid to weight loss. Hummus can help you stay on track because it contains both healthy fat and plant protein. When some fat is included in a meal, it causes us to feel full for longer.

One of my patients, Rosemarie, is the very fashionable wife of a prominent banker. She is known for her flair for entertaining, and is often compared to Martha Stewart. At her cocktail parties, Rosemarie often serves different varieties of healthy hummus with a selection of colorful crudités for the ladies, and a bowl of featherlight E.A.T. Olive Rosemary Thins from this famous Upper East Side gourmet grocery for the guys who are not watching their waistlines.

Be creative and add other ingredients to the recipes below to suit your taste: Red peppers, jalapeños for something more zesty, black and green olives, and fresh dill are all great variations to try.

GARLIC HUMMUS

2 cloves garlic
1 (12-ounce) can chickpeas, rinsed and drained
2 tablespoons lemon juice
3 tablespoons first-press extra-virgin olive oil

1.   In a food processor, mince the garlic.
2.   Add chickpeas, lemon juice, and olive oil.
3.   Process until smooth.
4.   Store in the refrigerator.

SERVING SIZE: 36 G • CALORIES: 67 • TOTAL FAT: 4 G • SAT FAT: 0 • CHOL: 0
• SODIUM: 90 MG • CARBS: 7 G • FIBER: 1 G • SUGARS: 0 • PROTEIN: 2 G

TAHINI HUMMUS

Tahini is ground sesame seeds. It can be found in a Greek or Middle Eastern grocery store, or check your local supermarket in the ethnic food aisle.

1 (15-ounce) can organic garbanzo beans (chickpeas), rinsed
    and drained
3 tablespoons organic tahini
1 to 2 cloves garlic, minced*
1/4 cup finely chopped fresh parsley
2 tablespoons fresh lime juice
1 1/2 tablespoons extra-virgin olive oil
1/2 teaspoon ground cumin
1/4 teaspoon sea salt
1/2 teaspoon white pepper
3 teaspoons water
Lime slices and parsley springs, for garnish

1.   Chop the garbanzo beans in a food processor briefly.
2.   Add the remaining ingredients (through white pepper) and process until mixed thoroughly.
3.   Add the water, one teaspoon at a time, until a smooth consistency is achieved.
4.   Garnish with fresh lime slices and parsley sprigs.

*May use more or less garlic to taste.

5. Serve with fresh crudités.
6. Refrigerate unused portion up to 1 week.

SERVING SIZE: ¼ CUP • CALORIES: 130 • PROTEIN: 4 G • CALCIUM: 33 MG

The Main Course—How the Rich Eat Themselves Thin

Lauren is a thirty-five-year-old woman with an extraordinary smile and sparkling personality. When she first came to my office, besides wanting to lose weight, she complained of migraine headaches and acid reflux disease. Both of these conditions have strong nutritional components. I advised Lauren to follow the Klauer Plan of high protein, mainly in the form of fresh fish, and to consume small, frequent meals. Not only did this high-energy woman lose 50 pounds and become drop-dead gorgeous, she permanently got rid of her headaches and indigestion. She is an inspiration to all who know her and shows the power that we all have to change. The following three recipes were created by this gifted woman.

LAUREN'S MARINATED TUNA

½ cup low-sodium soy sauce
2 tablespoons wasabi mustard
3 tablespoons ginger juice
2 cloves garlic, minced
Freshly ground black pepper
2 (5-ounce) fresh tuna steaks*
Sesame seeds, for topping

*Fresh tuna should be firm and flavorful. Bigeye tuna is moist and clean-tasting, truly rich in texture. Its flavor is more like meat than fish. It should have a deep ruby red color, and is best grilled or sautéed. It should never be overcooked, and is usually served rare. Another good variety is yellowfin, which is a lean meat but firm, with a large flake. It has a definite flavor of its own but is not too fishy, and should have a red color varying from a dark burgundy to a pale red.

One of my patients sends his housekeeper to Katagiri, a Japanese grocer and specialty store on East Fifty-ninth Street, to buy him only fresh sushi-quality tuna. They personally pick the fish from the Fulton Fish Market daily.

1.   Mix all the marinade ingredients together and marinate the tuna steaks for 1 hour, turning once or twice. Keep the fish in the refrigerator while it soaks.

2.   Grill over hot coals or on an oven grill for 5 minutes each side, basting with the marinade from time to time. Top with sesame seeds. Serves 2.

SERVING SIZE: 163 G • CALORIES: 191 • TOTAL FAT: 6 G • SAT FAT: 1 G • CHOL: 32 MG • SODIUM: 2,175 MG • CARBS: 12 G • FIBER: 2 G • SUGARS: 2 G • PROTEIN: 24 G

Ginger is a root plant, or rhizome, which spreads underground. It is widely used for medicinal purposes in China and India. Ginger has antioxidant, antimigraine effects and promotes digestion. It is often used to prevent motion sickness. Always use fresh ginger root for your recipes, as its flavor is intense. Store the unused portion of the root in the vegetable bin of the refrigerator.

LAUREN'S BROILED SALMON

2 tablespoons low-sodium soy sauce
$1/4$ cup fresh lime juice or bottled lime juice (without preservatives or sweeteners)
3 tablespoons rice vinegar
1 teaspoon black sesame oil
1 tablespoon ginger juice
Freshly ground pepper
2 (5-ounce) fresh salmon steaks*

1.   Preheat broiler.
2.   Mix the marinade ingredients together and marinate the salmon, skin side up, for 10 minutes.

*Tips for cooking farmed salmon, when you are unable to get wild salmon:

• Trim the skin and the visible fat, as PCBs are stored in the fat portion.
• Prepare your salmon by grilling and broiling, to reduce a significant portion of fat.

3. Under a preheated broiler, broil the salmon, with the skin side down, for 15 minutes.

4. Toward the end of the cooking time, spoon some of the marinade over the fish and cook until glazed. Serves 2.

SERVING SIZE: 169 G • CALORIES: 244 • TOTAL FAT: 14 G • SAT FAT: 2 G • CHOL: 60 MG • SODIUM: 649 MG • CARBS: 7 G • FIBER: 1 G • SUGARS: 2 G • PROTEIN: 23 G

LAUREN'S PAN-GRILLED HALIBUTS

2 (5-ounce) halibut steaks
Drizzle of olive oil
Dash of black pepper
1 mango, peeled and chopped
1/4 cup fresh cilantro
Juice of 1 lime
1 red onion, finely chopped
1 jalapeño pepper, minced
1/4 teaspoon ground cumin

1. Preheat oven to 400°F. Rub the halibut with olive oil and freshly ground black pepper. Place in grill pan and bake at 400 degrees until done all the way through. You can test the fish by cutting through the thick middle portion and taking a look. If it is cooked all the way through, it should be removed from the oven or it will become overly dry.

2. While the fish is cooking, mix together the salsa ingredients.

3. Serve fish with the salsa ingredients alongside it.

SERVING SIZE: 272 G • SERVINGS: 2 • CALORIES: 191 • TOTAL FAT: 2 G • SAT FAT: 0 • CHOL: 27 MG • SODIUM: 51 MG • CARBS: 25 G • FIBER: 3 G • SUGARS: 18 G • PROTEIN: 19 G

BLACK SOYBEAN SALSA WITH COD

5 tablespoons Lime-Shoyu Vinaigrette (see page 188)
15 ounces black soybeans
20 ounces fresh Atlantic cod
1 teaspoon ground black pepper
1 clove garlic, mashed
1 pound organic red tomatoes, chopped
½ cup sliced red onion
1 jalapeño pepper, chopped
2 tablespoons lime juice, plus extra to taste
Dash of salt to taste
Cilantro and lemon wedges, for garnish

1. In a large bowl, mix 3 tablespoons of the vinaigrette and the soy-
    beans. Cover and marinate in the refrigerator for at least 3 hours
    and preferably overnight. Stir occasionally.
2. Shortly before serving, cut the cod into four 5-ounce pieces. Brush
    both sides with the remaining 2 tablespoons of vinaigrette and dust
    with fresh ground black pepper. Set aside.
3. Toss garlic, tomatoes, onion, jalapeño, and lime juice with the mari-
    nated black soybeans and any unabsorbed marinade, adding extra
    lime juice and a dash of salt to taste, enough to give the mixture an
    edge. Using a slotted spoon, place about ¾ cup of the salsa in the
    center of each 4 plates.
4. Heat a large nonstick skillet over high heat. Sauté the cod until
    both sides are browned and the fish is no longer translucent in the
    center, 3 to 4 minutes per side. (If both sides are quite browned and
    the center is still raw, cover the skillet for the final minute or two of
    cooking, but make sure not to overcook.)
5. Serve with 6 ounces per serving of black bean salsa. Garnish with
    cilantro and lime wedges. Serves 4.

SERVING SIZE: 5 OUNCES • CALORIES: 540 • TOTAL FAT: 28 G • CHOL: 68.8 MG
• CARBS: 28.8 G • PROTEIN: 43.3 G

GREEK LAMB MEATBALLS WITH YOGURT TAHINI SAUCE

2 slices whole wheat bread
¼ cup fat-free milk
½ pound organic lamb shoulder or loin chop, trimmed of fat,
    ground*
1 tablespoon water
2 teaspoons fresh thyme
2 teaspoons fresh marjoram
½ teaspoon ground cinnamon
¼ teaspoon ground cardamom
¼ tsp. salt
Freshly ground black pepper to taste
1 tablespoon olive oil
Yogurt Tahini Sauce (optional, see page 198)

1. Cut bread into small pieces. Place on cookie sheets and dry overnight.
2. In a food processor, grind the dry bread pieces to crumbs. Combine the bread crumbs and milk using a fork.
3. Add the lamb and water to the bread crumbs, using your hands to combine. Add the herbs and spices and work until the mixture seems evenly combined.
4. Create 24 round meatballs, about 1 tablespoon each.
5. Heat the olive oil in a large nonstick skillet over medium-high heat. Cook, turning until all sides are evenly browned, about 5 to 7 minutes total.
6. Remove with a slotted spoon to a plate lined with a paper towel. Drain excess oil.
7. Serve immediately, with yogurt tahini sauce (recipe follows) if desired. Makes 24 servings.

MEATBALL ALONE

SERVING SIZE: 1 MEATBALL (ABOUT ½ OUNCE) • CALORIES: 32 • SAT FAT: <1 G • PROTEIN: 3 G • FIBER: 1 G • CALCIUM: 3 MG • CARBS: 1 G

*You may substitute lean ground beef, turkey chicken, or pork in place of lamb, or use a combination, if desired.

MEATBALL WITH TAHINI YOGURT SAUCE

SERVING SIZE: 1 MEATBALL + 1 TEASPOON SAUCE • CALORIES: 63 • SAT FAT: 1 G
  • PROTEIN: 4 G • FIBER: 1 G • CALCIUM: 15 MG • CARBS: 3 G

YOGURT TAHINI SAUCE

$^1/_2$ cup raw tahini
2 cloves garlic, minced
$^1/_2$ cup low-fat plain yogurt
$^1/_2$ cup freshly squeezed lemon juice

1.   In a medium-size bowl, add the garlic to the tahini.
2.   Slowly whisk in the yogurt and the lemon juice. Makes 74 teaspoon-size servings.

SERVING SIZE: 1 TEASPOON • CALORIES: 31 • PROTEIN: 1 G • SAT FAT: <1 G •
FIBER: 1 G • CALCIUM: 12 MG • CARBS: 2 G

SPAGHETTI SQUASH PARMESAN
WITH VEGETABLES

1 cup baked or boiled spaghetti squash
$^1/_2$ cup chopped spinach, steamed
$^1/_2$ cup red bell pepper, chopped
Kosher salt and black pepper to taste
$^1/_2$ cup pomodoro or marinara sauce (look for all-natural)*
$^1/_4$ cup part-skim mozzarella cheese

*In New York, we are blessed with a virtual explosion of high-quality food shops where you can get anything you want from anywhere in the world. One of my favorites is Agata & Valentina, on East Seventy-ninth Street. The minute you walk inside, one whiff sweeps you away to the villas of Tuscany. Their sauces are fresh and simple, and taste like they came out of an Italian grandma's kitchen. For the pomodoro sauce, rich red tomatoes are simmered with onions, roasted garlic, thyme, and oregano. You can make it your own by adding some of your favorite sautéed vegetables, or browned ground beef or turkey. These sauces are surprisingly low in fat, too: only about 2 grams per half-cup serving, and about 75 calories.

1. Preheat oven to 400°F.
2. Combined cooked squash, spinach, and bell pepper.
3. Sprinkle with kosher salt and black pepper to taste.
4. Place in an 8-inch square baking dish.
5. Cover with the sauce and bake in the preheated oven for 15 minutes.
6. Sprinkle with mozzarella cheese and place in oven until melted.
7. Remove and eat. Serves 2.

SERVING SIZE: 1 CUP • CALORIES: 106 • TOTAL FAT: 4 G • SAT FAT: 1.8 G • CHOL: 7.5 G • CARBS: 12.5 G • PROTEIN: 7 G

CHICKEN TENDERS

The secret to these tasty chicken fingers is the panko bread crumbs, which are imported from Japan, and can be found at Whole Foods and other specialty stores. These bread crumbs make an exceptionally delicate golden crust for all breaded dishes, and a terrific alternative to battered and deep-fried foods. For variety, serve chicken tenders on top of salad, or with broccoli, spinach, or spaghetti squash primavera Parmesan.

1 egg
4 ounces boneless, skinless chicken breast
¼ cup panko bread crumbs
Non-fat cooking spray

1. Beat egg.
2. Dip chicken in the beaten egg, then coat with panko crumbs.
3. Spray a nonstick grill pan, and heat over medium heat.
4. Cook the chicken for about 4 minutes on each side (depending on thickness of breast), until cooked.

SERVING SIZE: 1 (4-OUNCE) CHICKEN BREAST • CALORIES: 9 G • TOTAL FAT: 8 G • SAT FAT: 2.5 G • CHOL: 285 MG • CARBS: 9 G • OMEGA-3: 225 MG

VEGETARIAN CILANTRO CHILI

1 tablespoon extra-virgin olive oil
2 teaspoons minced garlic
1 1/2 cups diced onion
1/2 cup diced organic red bell pepper
1/2 cup diced organic orange bell pepper
1 teaspoon paprika
1 teaspoon ground cumin
1 1/2 teaspoons chile powder
1/2 teaspoon cayenne pepper
2 tablespoons low-sodium tamari
1 (15-ounce) can kidney beans
8 ounces canned organic soybeans
8 ounces canned organic white beans
1 (28-ounce) can crushed tomatoes
1 (28-ounce) can whole tomatoes
1 cup dry textured soy protein
1 cup water
2 tablespoons chopped fresh basil
2 tablespoons chopped fresh cilantro
1 1/4 cups low-fat mozzarella cheese, shredded

1. Heat the olive oil in a large Dutch oven over medium heat.
2. Add the garlic and onion, sautéing for about 3 minutes.
3. Add the red and orange bell pepper, sautéing another 1 to 2 minutes.
4. Add the paprika, cumin, chile powder, and cayenne pepper. Sauté about 30 seconds.
5. Add the tamari and all of the beans and tomatoes (with juice). Stir until well combined.
6. Add the textured soy protein and water. Stir well and simmer 20 to 30 minutes.
7. Remove the chili from heat and add the basil and cilantro. Stir to combine.

8. Ladle into bowls, sprinkle ½ ounce (⅛ cup) low-fat mozzarella cheese over the top of each bowl of chili. Serves 10.

SERVING SIZE: ½ CUP • CALORIES: 200 • PROTEIN: 16 G • CALCIUM: 208 MG

MEDITERRANEAN SHRIMP

The Mediterranean diet is one of the healthiest diets in the world. It relies on vegetables, herbs, fish, and olive oil. You can prepare this dish in five minutes, and it is absolutely delicious served alongside broccoli rabe or cooked spinach.

1 tablespoon olive oil
1½ pounds medium-size shrimp
Dash of salt and ½ teaspoon freshly ground black pepper
4 ripe tomatoes, chopped
3 cloves fresh garlic, minced
½ cup sun-dried tomatoes, rehydrated by soaking in hot water,
    drained and chopped
3 tablespoons capers
8 anchovy fillets, finely chopped
2 tablespoons fresh parsley, chopped
Handful of fresh basil, chopped

1. In a nonstick pan, heat the olive oil. When it is hot, add the shrimp, sprinkle with salt and pepper, and cook for 2 to 3 minutes on one side, then turn and cook for the same time on the other side. The idea is to have the oil hot and to not overcook the shrimp. Overcooking results in the shrimp becoming rubbery in texture. Transfer to a platter.
2. Add the tomatoes and remaining ingredients to the pan and simmer until tomatoes are tender and the flavors are blended. Return the shrimp to the pan and toss well to combine. Serve immediately. Serves 4.

SERVING SIZE: 272 G • CALORIES: 168 • TOTAL FAT: 6 G • SAT FAT: 1 G • CHOL: 102 MG • SODIUM: 726 MG • CARBS: 13 G • FIBER: 3 G • SUGARS: 7 G • PROTEIN: 18 G

SHRIMP AND BAKED TOFU SKEWERS

Whoever said skewers had to be boring metallic spears? This recipe utilizes aromatic rosemary branches. These are made by Jacob's Farm and can be found at www.wholefoodsmarket.com. The presentation of the dish is absolutely beautiful and could grace the fanciest dinner party. Preparation is surprisingly fast and easy.

1 package extra-firm tofu
2 tablespoons minced garlic
3/4 cup plus 4 tablespoons balsamic vinegar
2 tablespoons chopped fresh dill
2 tablespoons minced fresh ginger
1 lemon
10 large shrimp, peeled and deveined
4 rosemary skewers

1. Preheat oven to 350°F.
2. Cut the tofu into 1-inch cubes.
3. Mix together the garlic and the 4 tablespoons of balsamic vinegar, and marinate the tofu for 30 minutes.
4. Mix together the 3/4 cup balsamic vinegar, dill, and ginger.
5. On the skewers, alternate shrimp and pieces of tofu. Baste with the vinegar mixture. Cook in the preheated oven for 20 minutes, basting with the vinegar mixture. Squeeze a lemon over the kebabs just before serving.

SERVING SIZE: 398 G • SERVINGS: 2 • CALORIES: 179 • TOTAL FAT: 5 G • SAT FAT: 1 G • CHOL: 46 MG • SODIUM: 180 MG • CARBS: 15 G • FIBER: 1 G • SUGARS: 9 G • PROTEIN: 22 G

Lunch and Munch: Side Dishes

The more vegetables that you consume, the better! Vegetables should be the first thing that you reach for when you feel the need to "crunch." They are beautifully appetizing in appearance, have major health benefits, and are loaded with antioxidants.

LOW-FAT ASPARAGUS CHEESE SOUFFLÉ

2 cups chopped asparagus tips (you can substitute broccoli or
     spinach)
1/2 finely chopped onion
2 tablespoons olive oil
1 cup skim milk
3 tablespoons whole wheat flour
4 egg yolks (use omega-3 eggs)
2/3 cup grated low-fat Swiss cheese
Salt and fresh ground pepper
1/8 teaspoon ground nutmeg
6 egg whites
Pinch cream of tartar

1. Preheat oven to 425°. Butter a 1-quart soufflé dish.
2. Cook asparagus tips until tender but not mushy. When cool, drain and puree in a food processor.
3. In a heavy saucepan, sauté the onion in olive oil until tender.
4. In another saucepan, bring the milk to a boil. Meanwhile, sprinkle the flour over the cooking onion and stir constantly for 5 minutes. Turn off the heat and pour the boiling milk over the onion mixture while briskly whisking. Return to medium heat, and bring to boil while stirring constantly for 5 minutes.
5. Remove from heat. Stir in the egg yolks, one at a time. Then stir in the asparagus puree, grated cheese, salt, pepper, and nutmeg.
6. Beat the egg whites until foamy, add the cream of tartar, and continue to beat until stiff peaks are formed.
7. Take one-third of the egg whites and stir into the asparagus mixture. Then fold the remaining egg whites into the mixture. Do not overmix; you want this to be frothy, as this is what gives the soufflé its lightness.
8. Pour the mixture into the buttered soufflé dish and set into the pre-

heated oven. Reduce the heat to 375 degrees. You may check the soufflé after 20 minutes, it should have risen 2 inches from the rim of the dish and it should be browning nicely.

9.   Let it bake for 15 to 20 minutes more. Serve immediately. Makes 3 main-course portions.

SERVING SIZE: 365 G • CALORIES: 335 • TOTAL FAT: 18 G • SAT FAT: 5 G •
CHOL: 293 MG • SODIUM: 247 MG • CARBS: 18 G • FIBER: 3 G • SUGARS: 7 G
• PROTEIN: 28 G

GRILLED PORTOBELLO MUSHROOMS WITH GINGER

Portobello mushrooms are rich in iron, niacin, and selenium. Served alone, they are hearty enough to be a meal in themselves. They are also a wonderful accompaniment to simple grilled foods, such as fresh fish or chicken breasts.

4 portobello mushrooms
¼ cup balsamic vinegar
¼ cup orange juice
2 tablespoons ginger juice
3 tablespoons olive oil
2 tablespoons grated fresh ginger
Nonstick cooking spray
Lettuce, shredded, fresh basil, and fresh ginger, for serving

1.   Clean the mushrooms by thoroughly wiping with a damp paper towel. (Do not wash the mushrooms as they are like sponges and will soak up any water!) In a flat glass dish, place them stemless side up.
2.   Mix together the liquid ingredients and ginger, and pour over the mushrooms. Marinate in the refrigerator for 1 hour.
3.   Spray grill with nonstick spray. Grill the mushrooms over medium heat about 5 minutes on each side, turning occasionally. Serve on a lettuce leaf, topped with shredded basil and fresh ginger. Serves 4.

SERVING SIZE: 98 G • CALORIES: 130 • TOTAL FAT: 11 G • SAT FAT: 1 G •
CHOL: 0 • SODIUM: 5 MG • CARBS: 9 G • FIBER: 1 G • SUGARS: 3 G •
PROTEIN: 2 G

STEAMED SNOW PEAS WITH GARLIC AND GINGER

Snow pea shoots are lacy tendrils that surround the pea pod. They are delicate and delicious, and may be eaten in a salad or quickly cooked in hot oil and served as a vegetable. Pea shoots are low in calories, high in vitamins and minerals, and contain disease-fighting phytochemicals. Surprise your taste buds with this new treat!

1½ pound pea shoots, rinsed
2 cloves garlic, minced
2 teaspoons ginger juice
1 teaspoon low-sodium soy sauce

1. Place pea shoots and minced garlic in a steamer basket over boiling water.
2. Steam for 3 to 5 minutes.
3. Toss with the ginger juice and soy sauce. Serves 2.

SERVING SIZE: 261 G • CALORIES: 129 • TOTAL FAT: 1 G • SAT FAT: 0 •
CHOL: 0 • SODIUM: 100 MG • CARBS: 24 G • FIBER: 7 G • SUGARS: 10 G •
PROTEIN: 8 G

Desserts

Who ever said a "diet" plan can't include sinful desserts!

BERRY BANANA SMOOTHIE

1 (5.3-ounce) container Fage Total 0% Greek yogurt
⅓ cup organic skim milk
½ medium-size organic banana
¼ cup organic raspberries*
¼ cup organic blueberries*
1 to 2 ice cubes (optional)*

*You may use frozen, unsweetened organic berries and eliminate the ice cubes.

1.   Place all ingredients in blender and process until smooth.
2.   Serve immediately. Serves 1.

SERVING SIZE: 12 OUNCES • CALORIES: 225 • PROTEIN: 20 G • CALCIUM: 465 MG

PUMPKIN GINGER SOUFFLÉ

Nonstick cooking spray
Sugar for dusting
$1/2$ cup skim milk
$1^1/2$ teaspoons cornstarch
$1^1/2$ teaspoons crystallized ginger, finely chopped
$3/8$ cup pumpkin cooked, pureed (not pumpkin pie mix)
$1/4$ teaspoon ground cinnamon
1 dash ground cloves
$1/4$ teaspoon vanilla extract (or scrape the inside out of $1/2$
        vanilla bean)
4 egg whites
$1^1/2$ teaspoons sugar

1.   Preheat oven to 375°F. Prepare ramekins by lightly spraying each
      with Pam or another pan coating, and dusting with sugar.
2.   Invert the ramekins and rap to dislodge any excess sugar.
3.   Stir the cornstarch into the cold milk and heat the mix slowly until
      it boils and thickens; add the chopped crystallized ginger and set
      aside to cool.
4.   Combine the pumpkin with the other spices and vanilla; stir into
      the thickened milk.
5.   In a separate bowl, whip the egg whites to a soft peak, adding the
      sugar while whisking.
6.   Fold the pumpkin mix into the egg whites until consistent in texture
      and color.
7.   Portion into the prepared ramekins, and bake for 15 to 20 minutes
      at 375°F. Serves 6.

SERVING SIZE: 1 SOUFFLÉ • CALORIES: 30 • FAT: TRACE • CHOL: TRACE •
SODIUM: 448 MG • FIBER: TRACE • CARBS: 4 G • PROTEIN: 3 G

HOT APPLE WITH CINNAMON

1 Red Delicious apple
1 teaspoon ground cinnamon
$1/2$ teaspoon fresh lemon juice

1. Preheat oven to 350°F. Core and quarter apple. Sprinkle with the cinnamon and lemon juice.
2. Place in oven 15 to 20 minutes at 350°F, or microwave on High for $1^1/2$ to 2 minutes.
3. Serve on plate and eat with fork and knife. Serves 1.

SERVING SIZE: 140 G • CALORIES: 78 • TOTAL FAT: 0.3 G • CHOL: 0 • SODIUM: 2 MG • CARBS: 20.9 G • PROTEIN: 0.4 G

BAKED PEARS WITH WALNUTS
AND FIGS

The rich flavor is a perfect ending to a fall or winter meal. Calimyrnas are the ne plus ultra of figs. Since they are extremely perishable, most of the Calimyrna crop is used for dried figs, confectionaries, and pastries. This dish may be prepared ahead and just popped into the oven as you are dining on the main course.

4 medium-size organic Anjou pears
Juice of $1/2$ lemon
$1/2$ cup chopped raw organic walnuts
4 organic Calimyrna figs, chopped
2 teaspoons cinnamon, plus more for sprinkling
$1/2$ cup organic apple juice
1 teaspoon ground cloves
2 teaspoons organic vanilla extract

1. Preheat oven to 350°F.
2. Peel and cut pears in half from stem to base. Core the pears, leaving the bottom intact.

3.   Place the pear halves in a baking pan.
4.   Sprinkle lemon juice over the pear halves.
5.   Combine the chopped walnuts and figs in bowl. Fill each pear half with the mixture.
6.   Sprinkle pear halves with about ¼ teaspoon cinnamon each.
7.   Pour the apple juice into baking pan around pears.
8.   Add the cloves and vanilla extract to the apple juice, and sprinkle with more cinnamon, to taste.
9.   Bake the pears for about 45 minutes, spooning the apple juice over the tops of pears 2 to 3 times during baking time.
10.   Remove the pears from oven and cool briefly. Serve warm. Serves 8.

SERVING SIZE: ½ PEAR   •   CALORIES: 153   •   PROTEIN: 2 G   •   CALCIUM: 50 MG

CHOCOLATE WALNUT TORTE
WITH RASPBERRY COULIS

This antioxidant-packed torte will please the palate. The crumb is exactly as it should be and the moisture is perfect. The "crust" is almost like a brownie. This torte is so yummy that it stands on its own, even without the coulis. The torte with raspberry coulis is perfect as a festive Valentine's Day dessert. It is guaranteed to cure even a chocoholic's craving!

Special equipment: 9" springform pan, paper towel, small food processor, electric mixer, rubber spatula, fine-mesh sieve.

¼ cup coarsely chopped walnuts, or ½ cup whole

Canola oil, to lightly coat baking pan.

¾ cup unsweetened cocoa powder

¾ cup whole wheat pastry flour (DO NOT use regular whole wheat flour)

1 tablespoon baking powder

2 large eggs (use omega-3 eggs)

2 large egg whites

1 teaspoon vanilla extract

¼ cup plus 2½ tablespoons Splenda (see note on page 210)

¼ cup plus 1 tablespoon granulated white sugar

½ cup canola oil

½ cup brewed espresso, cooled

¼ cup fat-free milk

1 pint fresh organic raspberries

1 teaspoon fresh lemon juice

1. Toast walnuts: Place walnuts in a dry skillet. Heat and stir over medium heat till the aroma of the nuts can be smelled—about 4 minutes. Remove from skillet and allow walnuts to cool. Coarsely grind in a food processor.

2. Preheat the oven to 350°F. Lightly coat the bottom and sides of 9-inch springform pan using a paper towel and canola oil.

3. Sift the cocoa, flour, and baking powder together into a large bowl. Whisk till combined.

4. Whisk the ground walnuts into the dry ingredients. Form a well in the center and set aside.

5. Using an electric mixer, beat the eggs, egg whites, and vanilla on medium-to-high speed until very light and fluffy—about 3 to 4 minutes. Beat in ¼ cup each of the sugar and Splenda, 1 tablespoon at a time; the mixture will thicken. Then turn mixer to low speed. Pour the oil, espresso, and milk into egg mixture in a slow, steady stream until incorporated.

6. Pour the egg mixture into the flour mixture. Gently fold the egg mixture into the flour mixture, using a spatula. Do not overmix. Pour into the prepared springform pan. Bake until the edges pull away from the sides of the pan and the center is set—about 35 minutes.

7. Cool the cake on a wire rack for at least 30 minutes. Meanwhile, prepare the coulis: Puree in a blender or food processor the raspberries, remaining Splenda, remaining sugar, and lemon juice. (Add drops of water as necessary to puree raspberries. Do not use over 1 teaspoon total of water.) Strain out the seeds from the puree through a fine-mesh sieve. You will need to use a rubber spatula to push the pulp through, leaving the seeds in the strainer.

8. Release sides of springform pan from the torte. Cut into 16 slices. Drizzle 1 tablespoon of coulis over each slice of torte. Makes 16 servings.

WITH COULIS

SERVING SIZE: 1/16 CAKE + 1 TABLESPOON COULIS • CALORIES: 135 • SAT FAT: 2 G • CARBS: 12 G • FIBER: 3 G • PROTEIN: 3 G • CALCIUM: 31 MG

WITHOUT COULIS

SERVING SIZE: 1/16 CAKE • CALORIES: 124 • SAT FAT: 2 G • CARBS: 9 G • FIBER: 2 G • PROTEIN: 3 G • CALCIUM: 28 MG

Note: A word about Splenda. Though I do not recommend processed or synthetic foods in general, this is a sugar substitute made from sucralose, which is even suitable for diabetics. It has no calories, and can be used in all foods and beverages, and even in baking without leaving a bitter aftertaste. Available in packets and in granular forms, and a 5-pound "baker's bag" that would last you for life. It's been very helpful to my patients who want to add sweetness to baked goods without adding calories. Visit www.splenda.com for more information.

STRAWBERRIES WITH BALSALMIC VINEGAR

Basil is in the mint family and balsamic vinegar is great with fruit. This recipe can be made with fruits other than strawberries, such as blueberries, cantaloupe, honeydew melon, or pineapple. I've included nutrition information on those in case anyone is interested in omitting the strawberries.

½ cup balsamic vinegar
¼ cup white wine
2 tablespoons Splenda
2 cups fresh strawberries, rinsed and sliced
¼ cup basil leaves thinly sliced
1 cup low-fat vanilla yogurt

1. To prepare the sauce, combine the balsamic vinegar, white wine, and Splenda in a small saucepan. Heat on high until the mixture is reduced by half, about 15 minutes. It will become syruplike.
2. Once reduced, allow the mixture to cool.
3. While sauce is cooling, rinse and mix the strawberries and basil together. Stir the yogurt into the reduced sauce.
4. To serve, scoop the berries into four dessert bowls and then top with the yogurt sauce. Makes 4 servings.

SERVING SIZE: ¼ CUP FRUIT + 3½ OUNCES YOGURT SAUCE

	CALORIES	SATURATED FAT (G)	PROTEIN (G)	FIBER (G)	CALCIUM (G)	CARBS (G)
Strawberries	91	0	3	3	116	18
Blueberries	109	0	3	2	110	23
Cantaloupe	97	0	3	1	114	19
Honeydew	98	0	3	1	110	21
Pineapple	107	0	3	2	111	22

ROMAN POACHED PEARS WITH PEPPERCORNS

This recipe is divine. The pears melt in your mouth and their taste is a refreshing surprise from regular poached pears. I was inspired by the poached pears I had in a charming little trattoria in New Haven, Connecticut, a few years ago. The recipe here is not as sugary as the original, adding complexity to the flavor.

1 1/2 cups red wine

1/2 cup water

1/2 cup balsamic vinegar

1/4 cup Splenda

2 tablespoons whole peppercorns

4 pears

1.   In a 4-quart pan, combine the wine, water, vinegar, Splenda, and peppercorns.
2.   Bring to a boil, then reduce the heat to allow mixture to simmer.
3.   Slice the pears into sixths or more, and core them, leaving skin on.
4.   Place the pears in the mixture and simmer. Pears should be completely covered with the poaching liquid. If they are not, add more water.
5.   Simmer till very tender. The flesh should give little or no resistance when pierced with fork or skewer. This may take up to 30 minutes.
6.   Remove the pears and place into four individual serving bowls or on a platter with a rim.
7.   Strain out the peppercorns from the liquid and discard them.
8.   Return the liquid to the heat and bring to a boil until it is reduced and thickened. Pour over the pears.
9.   Serve warm or at room temperature. Makes 4 servings.

SERVING SIZE: 1 PEAR + ABOUT 1/2 CUP SAUCE • CALORIES: 217 • SAT FAT: 0 • CARBS: 42 G • FIBER: 4 G • PROTEIN: 1 G • CALCIUM: 26 MG

YOGURT CHEESECAKE

This cheesecake tastes just like a classic Italian cheesecake. It is lovely drizzled with fresh berries, too.

Special Equipment: fine-mesh strainer, cheesecloth, paper towels, 8- to 9-inch springform pan, small food processor, rubber spatula, mixer, large pan, chef's knife, tall glass

1 cup yogurt cheese (reduced from 2 3-ounce containers plain
    low-fat yogurt; see instructions below)
8 ounces Neufchâtel (or low-fat cream cheese), at room
    temperature, cut into chunks
1 cup low-fat (1%) cottage cheese, drained in a fine-mesh
    strainer for 30 minutes
Canola, safflower, or sunflower oil, if not using a nonstick pan
$\frac{1}{4}$ cup granulated sugar*
4 teaspoons Splenda
$\frac{1}{4}$ cup all-purpose flour
4 large eggs
2 large egg whites
2 teaspoons vanilla extract

1. To make yogurt cheese, place 2 (8-ounce) containers of plain fat-free yogurt into a fine-mesh strainer lined with cheesecloth, or into doubled cheesecloth, and drain over a bowl. Cover and place in the refrigerator overnight, or at least 4 hours. The longer the yogurt is drained, the drier the cheesecake will be. The length of draining depends upon your preference—a creamy cheesecake or a drier cheesecake.

2. After making the yogurt cheese, remove the Neufchâtel cream cheese from the refrigerator. Cut into chunks and allow it to come to room temperature—about 30 minutes.

3. Strain the cottage cheese at this time, too, for 30 minutes.

4. Preheat the oven to 500°F. If not using a nonstick pan, wet a paper towel with oil and lightly oil the base and side of the springform pan. In order to bake the cake in water bath, take a wide sheet of aluminum foil and set the springform pan on top of the foil. Fold the foil up the sides of the pan. This is to keep water from seeping into the cake from the seam of the springform pan, when the pan is later placed inside the larger pan filled with water.

5. In food processor, process the cottage cheese until smooth, 2 to 3 minutes. After a minute or so, use a rubber spatula to scrape down

---

*If desired, you may replace the sugar and Splenda with $\frac{1}{3}$ cup Splenda. I believe, however, that the taste is better if you include some sugar.

the sides; finish processing. With a mixer (not a processor) cream together the processed cottage cheese, Neufchâtel, sugar, Splenda, and flour. Add the yogurt cheese to the cheese mixture and only briefly blend. Using a whisk, lightly beat the eggs and egg whites together. Use the rubber spatula to fold the eggs and vanilla into the cheese mixture until well combined.

6. Pour the mixture into the springform pan. Smooth top. Set into the larger pan and fill the latter with water halfway up the sides of the springform pan. Bake at 500°F for 10 minutes to brown the edges and top, then reduce the heat to 250°F for one hour. Turn oven off and allow the cake to cool in the oven with the door ajar for 30 minutes. (Use a wooden spoon or spatula to keep the door ajar if necessary.)

7. Cover and refrigerate overnight, or for at least 6 hours. This allows time for cheese flavors to blend.

8. When ready to serve, remove from the refrigerator and let stand at room temperature for 30 minutes to an hour before slicing. Run a small knife around the edge of the cake, pressing the blade against the pan to prevent cutting the cake. Carefully remove the side of the pan. Leave the cake on springform pan bottom to serve. Fill a tall glass with hot water.

9. Using a chef's knife dipped in the hot water and wiped clean between each slice, cut the cheesecake into eight slices.

10. If desired, top with ¼ cup of fresh berries.

MADE WITH ¼ CUP SUGAR AND 4 TEASPOONS SPLENDA

SERVING SIZE: ⅛ CAKE • CALORIES: 192 • SAT FAT: 5 G • CARBS: 13 G • FIBER: 0 • PROTEIN: 12 G • CALCIUM: 125 MG

MADE WITH ⅓ CUP SPLENDA

SERVING SIZE: ⅛ CAKE • CALORIES: 170 • SAT FAT: 5 G • CARBS: 7 G • FIBER: 0 • PROTEIN: 12 G • CALCIUM: 125 MG

	CALORIES	SATURATED FAT (G)	PROTEIN (G)	FIBER (G)	CALCIUM (MG)	CARBS (G)
Blueberries (¹/₄ cup)	21	0	0	1	2	5
Strawberries (¹/₄ cup)	11	0	0	1	5	3

BLUEBERRY THYME PIE WITH OATS-AND-ALMOND CRUST

1 cup rolled oats
10 almonds
1 cup brown rice flour
¹/₄ teaspoon salt
1 tablespoon Sucanat (same as brown sugar) or Splenda
2 tablespoons sesame oil or 1¹/₂ tablespoons of applesauce
²/₃ cup ice water
4 cups fresh or frozen blueberries
2 tablespoons granulated sugar
¹/₂ cup fresh thyme—use leaves and buds, discard stems
3 tablespoons freshly squeezed lemon juice
2 tablespoons whole wheat pastry flour

1. Preheat oven to 350°F. To form crust, blend oats and almonds in dry blender to flour consistency, and place in a bowl. Combine with brown rice flour, salt, and Sucanat or Splenda. Add sesame oil or applesauce and stir; add water and mix to soft dough.
2. Press mixture into lightly sprayed pan, from center outward; crimp edges with fork or dampened fingertips. Prebake 10–15 minutes; when you take out the crust, set the oven to 400°F.
3. If using frozen blueberries, microwave in large microwaveable bowl on high for 5 minutes. Stir the frozen berries and continue to microwave for 2 to 3 more minutes, until their juices flow. If using fresh blueberries, microwave for 3 to 5 minutes total.

4.   Add the sugar, thyme, juice, and flour and mix. The mixture should be warm. If it is not, microwave 1 to 2 minutes.
5.   Pour into crust and bake until pie is bubbly and appears set, about 40 minutes. Or, bake in an 8-inch square pan without pastry.
6.   Use a crust guard toward end of baking (after about 30 minutes of baking) if necessary, to prevent crust from overbrowning.
7.   Remove from oven and allow to cool on a wire rack.
8.   Serve warm. Serves 8.

Nutritional information for pie with crust, if substituted Splenda and apple sauce:

SERVING SIZE: ⅛ PIE • CALORIES: 119 • TOTAL FAT: 2 G • SAT FAT: 0 • CHOL: 0
  • SODIUM: 75 MG • CARBS: 23 G • FIBER: 2 G • SUGARS: 1 G • PROTEIN: 3 G

Nutritional information for crustless pie baked in an 8 x 8-inch dish and divided into 9 portions:

SERVING SIZE: ⅑ PIE • CALORIES: 43 • SAT FAT: 0 • CARBS: 11 G • FIBER: 2 G
  • CALCIUM: 1 MG • PROTEIN: 1 G

SUBSTITUTIONS

• In recipes, replacing half the sugar with Splenda makes a tasty product. When baking entirely with Splenda, there may be an aftertaste.
• Canola vs. sunflower and safflower oils—these three oils can be used interchangeably in baking because they are so mild tasting. Canola has omega-3 but needs to be bought in an opaque container, otherwise omega-3 is lost. Canola is lowest in saturated fat of all the vegetable oils.

SILKY ALMOND SPREAD

This light and sweet spread is wonderful served with sliced apples or pears as a snack, for a simple dessert or even for lunch.

5 ounces raw whole organic almonds
6 ounces "lite" silken tofu
1/2 teaspoon ground cinnamon
1 teaspoon vanilla extract
2 tablespoons Splenda

1. Place almonds in food processor for approximately 7 to 10 minutes until smooth consistency is achieved.
2. Add remaining ingredients and process until mixed thoroughly.
3. Refrigerate unused portion up to 1 week. Yields 16 1-tablespoon servings.

SERVING SIZE: 1 TABLESPOON • CALORIES: 57 • PROTEIN: 3 G • CALCIUM: 62 MG

CANDIED PUMPKIN SEEDS

This is a really crunchy treat that takes only 20 minutes to whip up.

Canola, safflower, or sunflower oil
2 tablespoons granulated sugar
2 tablespoons Splenda
1/2 teaspoon ground cinnamon
1/2 teaspoon ground ginger
1 medium-size egg white
1/2 teaspoon freshly grated ginger
2 cups raw, unsalted pumpkin seeds

1. Preheat oven to 350°F.
2. Wet a paper towel with oil and lightly grease pan.
3. Whisk together the sugar, Splenda, cinnamon, and ginger.

4.   Beat the egg white till foamy in a medium-size bowl.
5.   Add the dry ingredients and fresh ginger to the egg white and thoroughly combine.
6.   Spread the seeds in a single layer on a baking sheet with sides.
7.   Bake until golden brown, stirring occasionally, for about 15 minutes.
8.   Remove from the oven and allow time to cool.
9.   Makes 8 servings. Keep leftovers in airtight container.

SERVING SIZE: ¼ CUP • CALORIES: 193 • SAT FAT: 4 G • CARBS: 4 G • FIBER:
3 G • PROTEIN: 9 G • CALCIUM: 20 MG

CHEWY GINGER BARS

Canola, sunflower, or safflower oil
½ cup whole wheat pastry flour
½ cup whole wheat flour
2 tablespoons granulated sugar
2 tablespoons Splenda
½ teaspoon baking soda
3 tablespoons minced, fresh ginger
¼ cup fat-free milk
¼ cup light molasses
2 large egg whites
1 tablespoon powdered sugar, if desired

1.   Preheat oven to 350°F.
2.   Lightly coat an 8-inch square glass baking pan with oil.
3.   In a large bowl, stir together the flours, sugar, Splenda, baking soda, and ginger.
4.   Whisk in the milk, molasses, and egg whites until well blended.
5.   Pour the batter into the prepared pan. Bake until the center springs back when lightly pressed, about 20 minutes.
6.   Serve warm. If desired, sprinkle on 1 tablespoon powdered sugar through a sieve or sifter. Makes sixteen 2-inch-square bars.

WITHOUT POWDERED SUGAR

SERVING SIZE: 2-INCH SQUARE • CALORIES: 46 • SAT FAT: 0 • CARBS: 11 G •
FIBER: 1 G • PROTEIN: 1 G • CALCIUM: 17 MG

WITH POWDERED SUGAR

SERVING SIZE: 2-INCH SQUARE • CALORIES: 48 • SAT FAT: 0 • CARBS: 11 G •
FIBER: 1 G • PROTEIN: 1 G • CALCIUM: 17 MG

RED, WHITE, AND BLUE PARFAIT

This is great for breakfast, too!

1 (5.3 ounce) container 0% fat Greek yogurt
1/4 cup fresh blueberries
1/4 cup sliced strawberries
1 teaspoon honey (optional)
1/4 cup crushed almonds*

1. Use a parfait dish.
2. Place a layer of yogurt on the bottom.
3. Add a layer of blueberries.
4. Top with another layer of yogurt.
5. Add a layer of sliced strawberries.
6. Add a dollop of yogurt on top.
7. Sprinkle with crushed almonds.

SERVING SIZE: 1 • CALORIES: 300 • TOTAL FAT: 14 G • SAT FAT: 1 G •
CHOL: 0 • CARBS: 28 G • PROTEIN: 22 G

*Calories and fat can be lowered by reducing the amount of almonds.

RICOTTA CUSTARD

$1/2$ cup farmer cheese
$3/4$ cup ricotta cheese
$1/4$ cup Splenda
2 omega-3 eggs
1 egg white
$1/4$ cup skim milk
$1/2$ teaspoon vanilla or almond extract
Orange or lemon rind, finely chopped (optional)

1. Combine farmer cheese, ricotta, and Splenda, and mix well. Stir in skim milk.
2. Add the eggs and egg white, and beat until mixed well and smooth; add extract.
3. Place into three 8-ounce ramekins. Place the ramekins in a 13 × 9-inch baking dish and cover the bottom of the baking dish with 1 inch of water.
4. Serve warm. Garnish with orange or lemond rind, if desired. Makes 3 servings.

SERVING SIZE: 8 OUNCES • CALORIES: 231 • TOTAL FAT: 16 G • SAT FAT: 7 G • CHOL: 556 MG • CARBS: 9 G • PROTEIN: 21 G

LEMON CHIFFON MOUSSE

1 (.25-ounce) package unflavored sugar-free gelatin
$1/4$ cup cold water
4 omega-3 eggs, separated
1 cup baking Splenda
$1/2$ cup fresh lemon juice
$1/2$ teaspoon HalsoSalt, or salt substitute
1 tablespoon freshly grated lemon zest

1. Soften the gelatin in water for 5 minutes
2. Beat the egg yolks and add $1/2$ cup of Splenda, the lemon juice, and

the salt. Cook in the top of a double boiler, stirring constantly, until it is of custard consistency.

3. Add the grated lemon zest and softened gelatin, and stir until incorporated completely. Cool.

4. When mixture begins to get thick, whip the egg whites until stiff in a clean bowl, adding the remaining $1/2$ cup of Splenda while whipping.

5. Fold the egg whites into the custard. Spoon into custard cups.

6. Chill in refrigerator. Makes 12 servings.

SERVING SIZE: 1 CUP • CALORIES: 26 • TOTAL FAT: 1.5 G • SAT FAT: 0.5 G • MONOUNSATURATED FAT: 6 G • POLYUNSATURATED FAT: 0.5 G

*The Pièce de Résistance—Le Socia*Lite

Alexis is a twenty-six-year-old Park Avenue glamour girl, Harvard educated, elegant in her manners and taste. She is a young woman who truly has all the gifts! While in Paris she came across a restaurant in the Seventeenth Arrondisement that serves a fabulous light dessert that had become quite popular with the Parisian fashion set. Alexis told me that she watched with amazement as cake after cake was carried out of the little bistro, called Chez Cool, where it was created.

I have served it to my friends who all have loved it, and I present the recipe to you, as Alexis did to me. I think you will adore it. It is low in calories, high in calcium and protein, looks wonderful, and is absolutely delicious! To make it extra festive, puree some fresh berries, strain them, and drizzle the juice all around each serving.

There is a Williams-Sonoma store on Madison Avenue and Eighty-sixth Street, where I found the perfect fleur-de-lis cake pan ($29), France's royal emblem, to make Le Socia *Lite* the envy of your guests. The pan is a cast-aluminum mold with pretty detailing and an all-important nonstick coating. Order at www.williamssonoma.com.

Don't let its indulgently fluffy texture and sweet taste fool you—this cake takes all of three minutes to create and is amazingly low in calories, around 60 per serving!

LE SOCIA*LITE*

8 ounces Fromage Blanc cheese
$^1/_2$ vanilla bean
1 envelope unflavored powdered gelatin
    (or 4 gelatin sheets)
4 tablespoons and 1 cup (250 g) of water
Zest of one lemon
Zest of one orange
5 packages of Splenda
1 peach, peeled
1 cup neutral glaze
2 ounces (80 g) peach puree

1. Place the Fromage Blanc cheese in a mixer and whip until smooth. Scrape the vanilla bean seeds out of the vanilla pod and mix it with cheese.
2. Mix the gelatin powder with 2 tablespoons of water and set aside to rehydrate (or soak the gelatin sheets in a separate bowl of cold water).
3. Put the lemon and orange zest in a small bowl with 3 packages of Splenda. Boil 1 cup of water and pour over the Splenda mix to dissolve. While the water is still hot, mix it with the prepared gelatin (or squeeze the gelatin sheets into the heated water). Add the gelatin mix to the Fromage Blanc. It should be very liquid. Let the mix come to room temperature.
4. Cut off a thin slice from the peach and place it in the bottom of a dome-shaped mold. Put two remaining packages of Splenda and 2 tablespoons of water in a small pot and heat to dissolve. Cut the rest of the peach into large cubes and place it in the same pot, poaching it for a few minutes until the water has evaporated (about 3 minutes). Set aside to cool.
5. Put the cooled mousse mixture $^1/_2$ way into the prepared mold. Add the poached peaches. Cover the mold with the remaining mousse. Place in the refrigerator to set up.

6.   Carefully unmold the mousse and place it on a screen. Pour neutral glaze mixed with peach puree over the dome.

SERVING SIZE: 36 G • CALORIES: 59 • FAT: 0 • CHOL: 4 MG • SODIUM: 517 MG • CARBS: 5 G • FIBER: 0 • SUGARS: 3 G • PROTEIN: 9 G

GLOSSARY

Antioxidants: Enzymes or other organic substances, such as vitamin E, vitamin C, and beta-carotene, that are capable of counteracting the damaging effects of oxidation in tissue.

Calcium: An element taken in through the diet that is essential for a variety of bodily functions, such as neurotransmission, muscle contraction, and proper heart function. Key sources include dairy products, soy, and some green leafy vegetables.

Calorie: Measurement of energy. The technical definition is: a unit of measurement defined as the amount of energy it takes to raise the temperature of 1 g of water from 15 to 16 degrees Celsius (or 1/100th the amount of energy needed to raise the temperature of 1 g of water at one atmosphere pressure from 0 degrees C to 100 degrees C). Food calories are actually equal to 1,000 calories (1 food calorie = 1 kilocalorie).

Carbohydrate: One of the nutrients that supplies calories to the body. Carbohydrates are compounds composed of carbon, oxygen, and hydrogen, arranged as monosaccharides (simple sugars) or multiples of monosaccharides (polysaccharides or starches). Simple sugars and starches are rapidly absorbed and raise blood glucose. Fiber, when present, acts as a protective shield around the starch, slowing its digestion. Sources include grains, fruits, vegetables, nuts, legumes, and other plant foods. When completely broken down in the body, a gram of carbohydrate yields about 4 calories.

Cardiovascular Disease: Principally heart disease and stroke, the nation's leading killer for both men and women among all racial and ethnic groups.

Cortisol: A hormone produced by the adrenal gland, stimulates conversion of proteins to carbohydrates, raises blood sugar levels, and promotes glycogen storage in the liver. It is released in response to stress.

Endorphins: Neuotransmitters that give a feeling of euphoria; endorphins are released during sustained physical exercise.

Folic Acid: Part of the vitamin B complex, important for the health of the nervous and cardiovascular systems.

Ghrelin: The peptide hormone released from the stomach, which signals hunger to the brain.

HDL Cholesterol: High-density lipoprotein cholesterol (the "good" cholesterol). The goal is for HDL to be greater than 65 for a female and 55 for a male. HDL cholesterol is protective against cardiovascular disease.

Hypertension: Hypertension is another name for high blood pressure. It is defined as a blood pressure of 140/90; prehypertension is 130 to 139/90; normal blood pressure is 120/90 or less. The presence of hypertension means the heart must work harder to pump blood into the circulatory system. Hypertension is a risk factor for cardiovascular disease.

Insulin: A polypeptide hormone secreted by the cells of the pancreas in response to high blood sugar levels, it controls the blood glucose level. Defective secretion of insulin is the cause of diabetes.

LDL Cholesterol: Low-density lipoprotein cholesterol (the "bad" cholesterol), LDL cholesterol is responsible for the formation of plaque in the arteries. LDL cholesterol should be less than 130 mg/dl for an individual without cardiovascular risk factors, and less than 130 mg/dl for an individual who has had a heart attack.

Leptin: Hormone produced by fat cells, which signals to the brain how much fat is present within the body. Overweight individuals have higher amounts of leptin than do slim individuals. It is believed that during weight loss, falling leptin levels are partly responsible for the plateau that can occur in dieting.

Obesity: An increase in body weight beyond the limitation of skeletal and physical requirement, as the result of an excessive accumulation of fat in the body. Defined by a Body Mass Index (weight in kilograms divided by height in meters squared) of 30 or greater.

Omega-3 Fatty Acids: A class of fatty acids that have a double bond three carbons from the methyl moiety and play a role in lowering cholesterol and LDL levels. High amounts are found in fatty fish.

Organic: Any foods grown without the use of chemical fertilizers or pesticides, in soil made rich by composting and mulching. In animal products, this means no antibiotics or growth hormones are used.

Proteins: Complex organic compounds that contain carbon, hydrogen, oxygen, nitrogen, and usually sulphur, the characteristic element being nitrogen. Proteins, the principal constituents of the protoplasm of all cells, consist essentially of combinations of amino acids in peptide linkages. They serve as enzymes, structural elements, hormones, and immunoglobulins, and are involved in oxygen transport, muscle contraction, electron transport, and other activities throughout the body.

Saturated Fat: A fatty acid with all potential hydrogen binding sites filled (totally hydrogenated fat). Diets high in saturated fat increase the risk for atherosclerosis.

Serotonin: A neurotransmitter and hormone that is synthesized from the amino acid tryptophan, this regulates emotion, hunger, and sleep.

Soy: A member of the legume family, soybeans are the world's primary source of vegetable protein. Soy is low-fat, cholesterol free, lactose free, and is a good source of calcium.

Trans fat: Also referred to as trans-fatty acid, a fat that has been altered to a form that the body cannot digest. Examples include hydrogenated and partially hydrogenated oils created by a manufacturing process as well as fats that have been exposed to excessive heat by cooking.

Type 1 Diabetes: Also referred to as juvenile-onset diabetes. It is an autoimmune disease in which the body produces antibodies that destroy the beta cells of the pancreas. The underlying cause is usually genetic, and it is commonly treated with daily insulin dosing. Insulin is necessary for the body to properly utilize glucose: without it, blood sugar rises to dangerous levels and damage occurs throughout the body.

Type 2 Diabetes: Also referred to as adult-onset diabetes. In this case, excessive consumption of carbohydrates over an extended period of time puts stress on the pancreas, which is required to release massive amounts of insulin to maintain normal blood glucose. Over time the pancreas can no longer keep up with the demand. When blood glucose rises above 120 mg/dl, diabetes is said to be present. This is considered more common in middle-aged overweight individuals and usually treated by diet control, weight reduction, or oral hypoglycemic agents.

RESOURCES

Books

Crowley, Chris and Henry S. Lodge, M.D. *Younger Next Year*. New York: Workman Publishing, 2004.

Diuguid, Carol. *New York City Gourmet Marketplace*. Zagat Survey, 2005.

Dolkart, Andrew. *Touring the Upper East Side: Walks in Five Historic Districts*. New York Landmarks Conservancy, 1995.

Legato, Marianne, M.D. *Eve's Rib*. New York: Three Rivers Press, 2003.

Stoll, Andrew L., M.D. *The Omega-3 Connection*. New York: Simon and Schuster, 2002.

Walford, Roy, M.D. *The Anti-Aging Plan*. New York: Four Walls Eight Windows, 1995.

Willcox, Bradley, M.D., and Craig Willcox, Ph.D. *The Okinawa Program*. New York: Clarkson N. Potter, 2002.

Newsletters

There are many excellent newsletters that offer good information about health topics. I suggest that you subscribe to any or all of these to keep yourself updated on health news. I am a subscriber to the letters listed below and put out copies in my waiting room for my patients. These newsletters are all about taking charge of your health and being responsible for it. The more you can learn, the better.

Dr. Andrew Weil's Self-Healing Newsletter. Dr. Weil is a pioneer in integrative medicine with a very wide reach; his newsletter contains very interesting topics. Visit www.drweilselfhealing.com.

The Harvard Health Letter. Contains general health information of interest to men and women. There are articles on a variety of topics, such as: aging, alternative medicine, and exercise. Additionally, there are specific newsletters that may be subscribed to at additional cost: *Harvard Women's Health Watch, Harvard Men's Health Watch, Harvard Heart Letter,* and *Harvard Mental Health Letter.* Their Web site is www.health.harvard.edu.

Mayo Clinic Health Letter. Gives commonsense health advice. The Mayo Clinic has an extensive list of publications, including a beautifully illustrated cookbook. Great Web site: www.mayoclinic.com.

Nutrition Action Health Letter. Produced by the Center for Science in the Public Interest, this newsletter has interesting articles. It looks at products from a consumer interest point of view; recent subjects of articles included: lead in water, nutritional content of fast food, and diet books. My favorite feature is the charts that compare supermarket or restaurant items.

Tufts University Health and Nutrition Letter. Offers excellent nutritional advice and gives monthly recipes. Their Web site is www. healthletter.tufts.edu.

Food Suppliers

Meat

These Web sites list grass-fed organic foods only:

www.eatwild.com lists the producers of grass-fed beef in all fifty states.
www.eatwellguide.org gives a directory of naturally raised beef, dairy,
    and produce. They also have a handy directory of restaurants; you
    just type in your zip code.

If you find grass-fed beef too grainy for your taste, these sources will
give you a good alternative. The meat is carried at fine butcher shops
and top restaurants throughout the United States:

www.nimanranch.com
www.colemannatural.com
www.laurasleanbeef.com

Fish

Wild Alaskan salmon is lower in mercury than Atlantic salmon.
It is free of PCBs, which are cancer-causing contaminants found in
farmed salmon. I have found absolutely delicious products at www.
kasilofseafoods.com. They carry vacuum-packed frozen salmon fillets,
canned wild salmon (great for salads, comes as fresh or smoked salmon),
and red crabmeat. Everything is very well packaged and top quality.

MERCURY LEVELS IN COMMERCIAL FISH
AND SHELLFISH[1]

TABLE 1. FISH AND SHELLFISH WITH HIGHEST LEVELS OF MERCURY

SPECIES	MERCURY CONCENTRATION (PPM)					
	MEAN	MEDIAN	MIN.	MAX.	NO. OF SAMPLES	SOURCE OF DATA
Mackerel, king	0.73	NA	0.23	1.67	213	Gulf of Mexico Report 2000
Shark	0.99	0.83	ND	4.54	351	FDA Survey 1990–02
Swordfish	0.97	0.86	0.10	3.22	605	FDA Survey 1990–02
Tilefish (Gulf of Mexico)	1.45	NA	0.65	3.73	60	NMFS Report 1978

TABLE 2. FISH AND SHELLFISH WITH LOWEST LEVELS OF MERCURY

SPECIES	MERCURY CONCENTRATION (PPM)					
	MEAN	MEDIAN	MIN.	MAX.	NO. OF SAMPLES	SOURCE OF DATA
Anchovies	0.04	NA	ND	0.34	40	NMFS Report 1978
Butterfish	0.06	NA	ND	0.36	89	NMFS Report 1978

TABLE 2. FISH AND SHELLFISH WITH LOWEST LEVELS OF MERCURY

SPECIES	MERCURY CONCENTRATION (PPM)					
	MEAN	MEDIAN	MIN.	MAX.	NO. OF SAMPLES	SOURCE OF DATA
Catfish	0.05	ND	ND	0.31	22	FDA Survey 1990–02
Clams	ND	ND	ND	ND	6	FDA Survey 1990–02
Cod	0.11	0.10	ND	0.42	20	FDA Survey 1990–03
Crab[2]	0.06	ND	ND	0.61	59	FDA Survey 1990–02
Crawfish	0.03	0.03	ND	0.05	21	FDA Survey 1990–03
Croaker (Atlantic)	0.05	0.05	0.01	0.10	21	FDA Survey 1990–03
Flatfish[3]	0.05	0.04	ND	0.18	22	FDA Survey 1990–02
Haddock	0.03	0.04	ND	0.04	4	FDA Survey 1990–02
Hake	0.01	ND	ND	0.05	9	FDA Survey 1990–02
Herring	0.04	NA	ND	0.14	38	NMFS Report 1978
Jacksmelt	0.11	0.06	0.04	0.50	16	FDA Survey 1990–02
Lobster (Spiny)	0.09	0.14	ND	0.27	9	FDA Survey 1990–02

TABLE 2. FISH AND SHELLFISH WITH LOWEST LEVELS OF MERCURY

SPECIES	MERCURY CONCENTRATION (PPM)					
	MEAN	MEDIAN	MIN.	MAX.	NO. OF SAMPLES	SOURCE OF DATA
Mackerel, Atlantic (North Atlantic)	0.05	NA	0.02	0.16	80	NMFS Report 1978
Mackerel, chub (Pacific)	0.09	NA	0.03	0.19	30	NMFS Report 1978
Mullet	0.05	NA	ND	0.13	191	NMFS Report 1978
Oysters	ND	ND	ND	0.25	34	FDA Survey 1990–02
Perch, ocean	ND	ND	ND	0.03	6	FDA Survey 1990–02
Pickerel	ND	ND	ND	0.06	4	FDA Survey 1990–02
Pollock	0.06	ND	ND	0.78	37	FDA Survey 1990–02
Salmon (canned)	ND	ND	ND	ND	23	FDA Survey 1990–02
Salmon (fresh/ frozen)	0.01	ND	ND	0.19	34	FDA Survey 1990–02
Sardines	0.02	0.01	ND	0.04	22	FDA Survey 2002–03

TABLE 2. FISH AND SHELLFISH WITH LOWEST LEVELS OF MERCURY

SPECIES	MERCURY CONCENTRATION (PPM)					
	MEAN	MEDIAN	MIN.	MAX.	NO. OF SAMPLES	SOURCE OF DATA
Scallops	0.05	NA	ND	0.22	66	NMFS Report 1978
Shad (American)	0.07	NA	ND	0.22	59	NMFS Report 1978
Shrimp	ND	ND	ND	0.05	24	FDA Survey 1990–02
Squid	0.07	NA	ND	0.40	200	NMFS Report 1978
Tilapia	0.01	ND	ND	0.07	9	FDA Survey 1990–02
Trout (freshwater)	0.03	0.02	ND	0.13	17	FDA Survey 1990–03
Tuna (canned, light)	0.12	0.08	ND	0.85	131	FDA Survey 1990–03
Whitefish	0.07	0.05	ND	0.31	25	FDA Survey 1990–03
Whiting	ND	ND	ND	ND	2	FDA Survey 1990–02

TABLE 3. MERCURY LEVELS OF OTHER FISH AND SHELLFISH

SPECIES	MERCURY CONCENTRATION (PPM)					
	MEAN	MEDIAN	MIN.	MAX.	NO. OF SAMPLES	SOURCE OF DATA
Bass (saltwater)[4]	0.27	0.15	0.06	0.96	35	FDA Survey 1990–03
Bluefish	0.31	0.30	0.14	0.63	22	FDA Survey 2002–03
Buffalofish	0.19	0.14	0.05	0.43	4	FDA Survey 1990–02
Carp	0.14	0.14	0.01	0.27	2	FDA Survey 1990–02
Croaker, white (Pacific)	0.29	0.28	0.18	0.41	15	FDA Survey 1990–03
Grouper	0.55	0.44	0.07	1.21	22	FDA Survey 2002–03
Halibut	0.26	0.20	ND	1.52	32	FDA Survey 1990–02
Lobster (North American)	0.31	NA	0.05	1.31	88	NMFS Report 1978
Mackerel, Spanish (Gulf of Mexico)	0.45	NA	0.07	1.56	66	NMFS Report 1978
Mackerel, Spanish (S. Atlantic)	0.18	NA	0.05	0.73	43	NMFS Report 1978

The Country Hen
Free-roaming, organically fed chickens produce these eggs.

    PO Box 333
    Hubbardston, MA 01452
    (508) 928-5414
    www.countryhen.com

Eggland's Best

These chickens get feed that is free of animal products and hormones, and are certified kosher.

    Eggland's Best, Inc.
    King of Prussia, PA 19408
    (800) 922-3447
    www.eggland.com

Pilgrim's Pride EggsPlus

    PO Box 93
    Pittsburg, TX 75686
    800-824-1159
    info@pilgrimspride.com

Chino Valley Ranchers Organic Omega-3 Eggs

    5611 Peck Road
    Arcadia, CA 91006-5851
    (800) 354-4503

New York Eateries

These are some of my favorite New York restaurants that I recommend to my patients. In New York, there are more great restaurants than bad ones, but you have to choose wisely.

If you choose your dining experience wisely, you can stay on the Klauer Plan when entertaining lavishly for business dinners as well as dining out family style with your kids.

Atlantic Grill
A very popular seafood place, serving fresh sashimi and simply grilled fish, as you like it. They are famous for their filling Lobster Cobb Salad too.

> 1341 Third Avenue at Seventy-seventh Street
> 212-988-9200
> www.brguestrestaurants.com

Aureole
World-class American cuisine and fine dining, with a staff that are very eager to please, so special requests are the norm. Famous for their Simple Grills with a selection of portobello mushrooms, tuna, steak, chicken breast, salmon, and even pork served with herb-grilled vegetables. The Olive-oil Poached Alaskan Halibut with Fricassee of White and Green Asparagus is also splendid.

> 34 East Sixty-first Street
> 212-319-1660
> www.charliepalmer.com

Beppe
Wonderful Italian cooking, and they have their own organic farm in upstate New York. The Pontormo salad of field greens with scrambled eggs is a low-fat, high-protein treat.

> 45 East Twenty-second Street
> 212-982-8422

Better Burger
Fast food, the Upper East Side way, serving organic beef, lean turkey, and preservative-free hot dogs. Cheap and cheerful locations with delivery service.

1614 Second Avenue
212-734-6644
www.betterburgernyc.com

Brio
A perfect little Italian place to have a bite after a hard day of shopping at Bloomies.

786 Lexington Avenue at Sixty-first Street
212-980-2300

Café Boulud
Eclectic French cuisine in an intimate setting. Chef Boulud offers Le Potager Diner, a spring vegetarian menu. They also serve a wild Alaskan white salmon that is unique and delicious grilled.

20 East Seventy-sixth Street
212-772-2600
http://www.danielnyc.com/

Candle 79
Vegetarian dishes sure to please even diehard meat eaters. Start with their Hydrogarden Farm Edamame with Celtic Sea Salt. Tofu can be added to any of their salads for extra protein.

154 East Seventy-ninth Street
212-537-7179
http://www.candlecafe.com/

Coco Pazzo
Wonderful Italian cuisine that has become a traditional Upper East Sider's favorite. They respond to requests that no butter be used, and serve vegetables before dinner. Try the Poletto al Mattone, a wonderfully prepared chicken cooked with lemon and red pepper in a cast-iron skillet.

23 East Seventy-fourth Street
212-794-0205
www.cocopazzonewyork.com

Dock
A busy, popular seafood eatery in the heart of midtown. All their fresh fish can be simply grilled or broiled. Try the Seared Yellowfin Tuna or Pan-roasted Red Snapper, and substitute steamed broccoli for the baked potato.

> 633 Third Avenue
> 212-986-8080
> www.docksoysterbar.com

Esca
A wonderful place for fresh seafood dinners, right in the heart of the theater district. Their selection changes daily, based on what comes in from the fish markets. The Branzino (cod) and Rombo (roasted turbot) are always good.

> 402 West Forty-third Street
> 212-564-7272
> www.esca-nyc.com

Fred's at Barneys New York
The Mark Salad with tuna is excellent. Ask for a lower amount of olive oil than is provided. I order the same thing all the time there—Fred's Madison Salad with red leaf lettuce, beets, peas, and canned Italian tuna. The fruit plate is my favorite—it is always beautifully arranged with seasonal berries and melons. They also deliver!

> 660 Madison Avenue
> 212-833-2200

Gobo
Pan-Asian and Pacific Rim, vegetarian, and Japanese dishes full of flavor and fresh juices; and smoothies made with exotic ingredients like wolfberry and kumquat, to which you can add a boost of flaxseed for added benefit.

> 1426 Third Avenue at Eightieth Street
> 212-288-5099
> http://www.goborestaurant.com

Haru

Good, fresh, artfully prepared sushi. On weekends, the line extends down the block to get into this local hangout. There is a sexy bar across the street with the same owners, too, that serves great tartare: try the salmon tartare with citrus jalapeño sauce or yellowtail with sesame lemon sauce.

> 1329 Third Avenue
> 212-452-2230
> www.harusushi.com

Josie's

Featuring casual and healthy American vegetarian fare, the stir-fry entrées with tofu, chicken, calamari, and shrimp are lightly wok sautéed with canola oil, tamari, mirin, ginger, and garlic.

> 565 Third Avenue
> 212-490-1558
> www.josiesnyc.com

La Goulue

This is a favorite East Side destination spot among my patients, where you can easily run into people you know. In its early days, La Goulue entertained such femmes fatales as Jacqueline Onassis and Catherine Deneuve. You always have to make sure you are dressed to be seen when dining there, and the place is awash in Chanel suits and Kelly bags. They serve delicious bistro fare, but have the breadbasket removed. The tuna tartare with cilantro lime dressing is a must, but their crème brûlée is out.

> 764 Madison Avenue at Sixty-fourth Street
> 212-988-8169

Le Biblioquet

Chic, French, and lively bistro food. Don't be tempted by their superb French fries though; order the grilled fish and green salad. I get a kick out of the energy in that place! You can easily walk by this little jewel, as they do not even have a sign outside.

25 East Sixty-third Street
212-751-3036

Le Charlot
Owned by the same restaurateur as Le Biblioquet, this East Side bistro is another little bit of Euro heaven. Their roast chicken is satisfying, as is grilled sole minus the buttery sauces, or steak frites sans the frites.

19 East Sixty-ninth Street
212-794-1628

Orsay
This was formerly the site of the renowned Mortimer's, a gathering spot to be seen at in the 1980s, where New York's grand dames of the social world entertained their guests in the private room. It is now a French brasserie serving great salads, a dairyless vegetable soup, grilled meats, and wonderful tartares.

1057 Lexington Avenue at Seventy-fifth Street
212-517-6400
http://www.orsayrestaurant.com

Park Avenue Café
Clubby-style American cuisine with fresh seafood, such as Sauteed Jumbo Sea Scallops with Spaghetti Squash. They also have a vegetarian entrée called Tastings of Farm Harvest Vegetables that is perfect for the Klauer Plan. They have a special three-course "Pay Your Age Dinner" starting at 8:30 P.M., which can be a fun evening with friends. And the legendary Chopped Salad with feta cheese is a big hit with the "ladies who lunch" crowd.

100 East Sixty-third Street
212-644-1900
www.parkavenuecafe.com

Payard Patisserie
This chic French bistro offers beautifully prepared fish and vegetables. Order Dr. Klauer's Le Socia*Lite* for dessert!

1032 Lexington Avenue between Seventy-third and Seventy-fourth
  streets
212-717-5252
www.payard.com

Petrossian
The ultimate for true Russian caviar, fit for a czar! Beluga is the best
quality, produced from Beluga sturgeon. Their most exclusive variety is
the Imperial Special Reserve Persicus, available in limited quantities.
They also carry truffles, smoked white salmon, sturgeon sausages, and
other unique delicacies.

182 West Fifty-eighth Street
212-245-2214
www.petrossian.com

Primola
Authentic Italian cuisine in a cozy, intimate setting. I love this little place
and Giuliana, the manager, is always charming. I always have their sea
bass prepared Tuscan style with olives and tomatoes.

1226 Second Avenue at Sixty-fourth Street
212-758-1775

Swifty's
Very stylish but low key, this small and always crowded haven for the
Park Avenue crowd serves a lovely steamed artichoke vinaigrette, and
the *plus parfait* paper-thin chicken paillard with vegetables. They also
have their own private-label caviar for special patrons.

1007 Lexington Avenue
212-535-6000
www.swiftysny.com

Zen Palate
Asian-style vegetarian sanctuaries with several locations throughout
Manhattan. An ideal lunch for the first 3 days of the diet is the Kale and
Seaweed Salad served with tofu.

2170 Broadway
212-501-7768

Shop Till You Drop

My recommendations for time-saving New York City grocers at which to purchase healthy, whole foods that will help you stick with my plan!

Agata & Valentina
Italian gourmet shop featuring cheeses, meats, seafood, and fresh produce

1505 First Avenue
212-452-0690

Albert's Prime Meats
Old-world-style butcher shop featuring organic meats

836 Lexington Avenue
212-751-3169

A Matter of Health
Boasts a fresh-juice bar, healthy salads, and a plethora of vitamins

1478 First Avenue
212-288-8280

Balducci's
Runs the gamut of specialty and imported fresh foods

155 West Sixty-sixth Street
212-653-8320
www.suttongourmet.com

Baldwin Fish Market
Fresh fish brought in daily

1584 First Avenue
212-288-9032

A.L. Bazzini Co.
Gourmet market specializing in fresh nuts

339 Greenwich Street
212-334-1280

Butterfield Market
Landmark gourmet grocer

1114 Lexington Avenue
212-288-7800
www.butterfieldmarket.com

Caviarteria
The ultimate caviar emporium

1012 Lexington Avenue
212-759-7410
800-4-CAVIAR
www.caviarteria.com

Central Fish Co.
Fresh seafood at great prices

527 Ninth Avenue
212-279-2317

Citarella
Citarella is best known for its fresh seafood, with retail stores on the
East and West sides of Manhattan, delivery service, and online ordering.

1313 Third Avenue at Seventy-fifth Street
212-874-0383
866-248-2735
www.citarella.com

Dean & Deluca
One of the most sophisticated posh city grocers

>   1150 Madison Avenue at Eighty-fifth Street
>   212-717-0800
>   www.deandeluca.com

Zabar's
Zabar's is perhaps the most famous New York landmark for gourmet eating, and a longtime favorite with foodies as well as tourists.

>   2245 Broadway between Eightieth and Eighty-first streets
>   212-787-2000
>   www.zabars.com

Eli's
This group of upscale gourmet groceries is the Upper East Sider's playground.

Eli's Manhattan

>   1411 Third Avenue at Eightieth Street
>   212-717-8100

Eli's Vinegar Factory

>   431 East Ninety-first Street between First and York avenues
>   212-987-0885

E.A.T.
>   Most famous for a snack after a museum jaunt and for their decadent $45 Caviar Omelet
>
>   1064 Madison Avenue
>   212-772-0022
>   www.elizabar.com

Fairway

An Upper West Side institution, this fresh grocery carries a huge variety of produce, meats, and prepared dishes, with a second location in Harlem where my patients send their drivers to pick up cartons. No delivery service.

> 2127 Broadway and Seventy-fourth Street
> 212-595-1888
> www.fairwaymarket.com

Fresh Direct

A brilliant grocer that delivers all over the New York metro area, including the Hamptons. All New York doormen know when the Fresh Direct truck comes. They carry everything from organic fruits and vegetables, meats, fish, and seafood to bulk items, including waters and green tea. Their Web site is well designed and user friendly, and each product featured has full nutritional content, so you can stick with Dr. Klauer's plan with ease.

> www.freshdirect.com

Gourmet Garage

Specialty grocer

> 1245 Park Avenue
> 212-348-5950
> www.gourmetgarage.com

Grace's Marketplace

Shopping at Grace's Marketplace is best left to your housekeeper, who will sign for whatever you need on your house charge. If you see the prices, your blood pressure will surely shoot up!

> 1237 Third Avenue
> 212-737-0600
> 888-472-2371
> www.gracesmarketplace.com

Greenmarket
Seasonal outdoor farmer's market with locations all over Manhattan on
Sundays, year round. This is a perfect place to pick up organic vegetables
fresh from the farm, and delicious fresh-picked fruits. Plus, it's a fun
way to spend a Sunday morning.

> 212-477-3220
> www.cenyc.org

Hale and Hearty Soups
This Manhattan soup chain offers a delectable selection with healthy salads, too, a perfect spot for a quick lunch. They have locations throughout Manhattan.

> 212-517-7600

Health Nuts
Food store chain for the nutrition conscious and organic shopper

> 1208 Second Avenue
> 212-593-0116

Itoen Tea Store
An elegant Upper East Side oasis from one of Japan's largest tea merchants that carries a wonderful selection of green and white teas in beautiful packaging, nice enough to make a unique hostess gift. They have a
restaurant at their flagship store as well.

> 822 Madison Avenue at Sixty-eighth Street
> 1-888-697-8003
> www.itoen.com

Katagiri
Authentic Japanese specialty and grocery store

224 East Fifty-ninth Street
212-755-3566
www.katagiri.com

Leonard's
Fresh seafood, poultry, and meats suitable for entertaining

1385 Third Avenue
212-744-2600

Likitsakos
Greek and Mediterranean gourmet foods

1174 Lexington Avenue between Eightieth and Eighty-first streets
212-535-4300

Lobel's Prime Meats
This butcher is a cut above the rest, and carries great organic meats.

1096 Madison Avenue
212-737-1373
800-556-2357
www.lobels.com

Marché Madison
Grocery and prepared foods, with a good selection of yogurts, coffees, and teas

931 Madison Avenue at Seventy-fourth Street
212-794-3360

Natural Frontier
Health food grocer, stocked with organic vegetables and fruits

1424 Third Avenue
212-794-0922
www.naturalfrontiermarket.com

Ottomanelli Brothers
Traditional Italian butcher shop

> 1549 York Avenue
> 212-772-7900
> www.ottomanellibros.com

Peapod
National chain of supergrocers

> www.peapod.com

Pink Salmon
Great sushi

> 1163 Madison Avenue
> 212-535-7979

True Foods
A great source for natural and organic foods

> www.truefoodsmarket.com

Uptown Whole Foods
Wonderful selection of healthy goods

> 2421 Broadway
> 212-874-4000

Westerly Health Foods
A very down-to-earth grocer

> 913 Eighth Avenue
> 212-586-5262
> www.westerlynaturalmarket.com

Whole Foods
Chain of natural supermarkets with stores all over the country. I was so
excited when they opened in New York, too!

> 10 Columbus Circle
> 212-823-9600
> 888-746-7936
> www.wholefoodsmarket.com

William Poll
Sumptuous prepared foods, and smoked salmon to die for

> 1051 Lexington Avenue
> 212-288-0501
> 800-951-7655
> www.williampoll.com

NOTES

2. Protein—The Anchor of Your Diet

1. M. B. Schulze, J. E. Manson, D. S. Ludwig, et al., "Sugar-Sweetened Beverages, Weight Gain, and Incidence of Type 2 Diabetes in Young and Middle-Aged Women," *Journal of the American Medical Association* 292, no. 8 (2004): 927–34.
2. R. Covetti, M., Porrini, A. Santangelo, G. Testolin, "The Influence of the Thermic Effect of Food on Satiety," *European Journal of Clinical Nutrition* 52 (1998): 482–8.

3. Calcium—The Miracle Mineral

1. D. A. McCarron, C. D. Morris, C. Cole, "Dietary Calcium in Human Hypertension," *Science* 217 (1982): 267–9.

2. L. J. Appel, T. J. Moore, E. Obarzanek, et al., "A Clinical Trial of the Effects of Dietary Patterns on Blood Pressure," *New England Journal of Medicine* 336, no. 16 (1997): 1117–24.

3. K. Wu, W. C. Willett, C. S. Fuchs, et al., "Calcium Intake and Risk of Colon Cancer in Men and Women," *Journal of the National Cancer Institute* 94, no. 6 (March 20, 2002): 437–46.

4. P. R. Holt, "Dairy Foods and the Prevention of Colon Cancer: Human Studies," *Journal of American College of Nutrition* 199, no. 18 (5 Suppl.): 379S–91S.

5. B. Xue, A. G. Greenberg, F. B. Kraemer, M. B. Zemel, "Mechanism of Intracellular Calcium Inhibition of Lipolsis in Human Adipocytes," *FASEB Journal* 2110, 15:2, 527–9.

6. B. Eaton, D. A. Nelson, "Calcium in Evolutionary Perspective," *The American Journal of Clinical Nutrition* 54 (1991): 281S–7S.

7. M. B. Zemel, "Role of Calcium and Dairy Products in Energy Partitioning and Weight Management," *The American Journal of Clinical Nutrition* 79, no. 5 (May 2004): 907S–12S.

6. The Stop! Watch! Method of Exercise

1. W. Kemmler et al., "Benefits of 2 Years of Intense Exercise on Bone Density, Physical Fitness, and Blood Lipids in Early Postmenopausal Osteopenic Women: Results of the Erlangen Fitness Osteoporosis Prevention Study," *Archives of Internal Medicine* 164, no. 10 (May 24, 2004): 1084–91.

2. C. G. Mittleman, M. A. Kawachi I, et al., "Sexual Function in Men Older than 50 Years of Age: Results from the Health Professionals Follow Up Study," *Annals of Internal Medicine* 139, no. 3 (August 2003): 161–8.

7. Anti-Aging Nutrition: Live Longer and Look Younger

1. A. Benetos, K. Okuta, M. Lajemi, et al., "Telomere Length as an Indicator of Biological Aging: The Gender Effect and relation with Pulse Pressure and Pulse Wave Velocity," *Hypertension* 37, no. 2 (February 2001): 381–5.

2. E. Epel, E. Blackburn, et al., "Accelerated Telomere Shortening in Response to Life Stress," *PNAS* 101, no. 49 (December 7, 2004): 7312–5.

3. R. Walford, *The Anti-Aging Plan*, New York: Four Walls Eight Windows, 1995.

4. J. Victoroff, *Saving Your Brain: The Revolutionary Plan to Boost Brain Power, Improve Memory and Protect Yourself Against Aging and Alzheimer's*, New York: Bantam Press: 2002.

5. M. Hull, L. Lieb, B. L. Fiebich, "Pathways of Inflammatory Action in Alzheimer's Disease: Potential Targets for Disease Modifying Drugs," *Current Medical Chemistry* 9, no. 1 (January 2002): 83–8.

6. M. S. Apounder, C. R. Savage, D. Blazer, et al., "Predictors of Cognitive Change in Older Persons: MacArthur Studies of Successful Aging," *Psychological Aging* 10 (1995): 578–89.

7. D. E. Barnes, K. Yaffe, W. A. Santariano, et al., "A Longitudinal Study of Cardiorespiratory Fitness and Cognitive Function in Healthy Older Adults," *Journal of the American Geriatrics Society* 51, no. 4 (April 2003): 459–65.

8. D. Rudman, A. G. Feller, H. S. Nagraj, et al., "Effects of Human Growth Hormone in Men over 60 Years Old," *New England Journal of Medicine* 323, no. 1 (July 5, 1990): 1–6.

9. D. R. Taaffee, L. Pruitt, J. Reim, et al., "Effect of Recombinant Human Growth Hormone on the Muscle Strength Response to Resistance Exercise in Elderly Men," *Journal of Clinical Endocrinology and Metabolism* 79 (1994): 1361–6.

10. I. M. Lee, J. E. Manson, C. H. Hennekens, R. S. Paffenbarger, et al., "Body Weight and Mortality: A 27-Year Follow-up of Middle-aged Men," *Journal of the American Medical Association* 270 (1993): 2823–8.

11. J. E. Manson, W. C. Willett, M. J. Stamfer, et al., "Body Weight and Mortality Among Women," *New England Journal of Medicine* 333 (1995): 677–85.

12. B. Willcox and C. Willcox, *The Okinawa Program*, New York: Clarkson N. Potter, 2002.

8. Your Outside Is a Mirror of Your Inside

1. T. Perls and M. Silver, *Living to 100*, New York: Basic Books, 1999.
2. P. Lavie, "Sleep Disturbances in the Wake of Traumatic Events," *New England Journal of Medicine* 345, no. 25 (December 20, 2001): 1825–32.
3. Ibid.
4. R. C. Lavie, K. A. McGonagle, S. Zhao, et al., "Lifetime and 12-Month Prevalence of DSM-III-R Psychiatric Disorders in the United States: Results from the National Comorbity Survey," *Archives of General Psychiatry* 51 (1994): 8–19.
5. Ibid.
6. A. Lutz, L. L. Greischar, N. B. Rawlings, et al., "Long-term Mediators Self-Induce High Amplitude Gamma Synchrony During Mental Practice," *Proceedings of the National Academy of Sciences in the United States of America* 101, no. 46 (November 16, 2004): 16369–73.

INDEX